Contents

Health is not valued until sickness comes.

— Thomas Fuller

1. A Kernel of Truth: Understanding the Controversy

"Apricot Seeds for Cancer: A Dangerous Misinformation" is a meticulously researched, compelling exploration of how myths and misconceptions can deeply influence public health decisions. At first glance, the idea that something as humble as an apricot seed could potentially battle cancer seems almost magical, a natural remedy standing bravely in the face of one of humanity's most feared diseases. Yet beneath this appealing surface lies a web of misinformation, one that not only misguides but also endangers. As we set out on this enlightening journey, we will dissect the historical allure of natural cures, examine the rise of alternative medicine in an age of increasing scientific rigor, and unravel the tale of apricot seeds—claimed by some to be a cure, yet denounced by the scientific community as perilous. Join me, Isaac Frederick King, as we traverse the fascinating terrain of hope, science, deception, and health advocacy to uncover the true story behind this persistent myth.

2. The Historical Allure of Natural Cures

2.1. Ancient Remedies: A Glimpse into the Past

In exploring ancient remedies, particularly from the tenure of time before modern medicine, we are drawn into a world that revels in the harmony between nature and health. This paradigm, embedded in many cultures, prompts an examination of the ways in which our ancestors sought to heal and remedy ailments with minimal resources, tapping into their keen observations of the natural environment. Ancient remedies arose from a blend of spirituality, mysticism, and empirical trial and error, leading to a variety of natural treatments still in discussion today.

Historically, many societies turned to plants for healing, believing in their intrinsic connection to human health. The medicinal potential of herbs, roots, seeds, and flowers played a significant role in daily life, where shamans, herbalists, or wise women often held revered positions as healers. From the golden fields of ancient Egypt, where garlic was consumed for its health benefits, to the intricate pharmacopoeias of Traditional Chinese Medicine that incorporated thousands of plants, humanity's quest for wellness has been often entwined with a respect for the natural world.

In ancient Greece, the philosopher Hippocrates, often referred to as the father of medicine, laid the groundwork for herbal remedies, emphasizing the importance of diet and lifestyle in maintaining health. His belief that the body could heal itself led to the cultivation of various herbs, with plants such as willow bark, surpassing ancient times into modern use as aspirin. Ancient Indian texts like the Vedas cited over 1,000 plant species, establishing the foundations of Ayurveda, a holistic medical system that remains influential today.

Many of these remedies have transitioned into folk medicine, embodying the cultural heritage and accumulated wisdom of communities across the world. For instance, laurel leaves, anciently recognized for their anti-inflammatory properties, continue to be employed in cooking and herbal teas. Honey, as utilized by various cultures for its antibacterial properties, has persisted as a staple in both home remedies and commercial products. However, as is evident from the myriad of practices, not all historical remedies have withstood the scrutiny of modern science.

Specific to the narrative of apricot seeds, the early usage of their extracts might relate back to more rudimentary understandings of health and disease. The seeds, or kernels, of apricots were likely consumed in regions where the fruit thrived, and the allure of the seed's potential health benefits grew alongside folklore. Stories of the seeds' curative properties were likely fostered by the particular conditions under which they were consumed—perhaps alongside a diet rich in fruits and vegetables or within a community that emphasized holistic, natural health practices.

Despite their traditional usages, ancient remedies present a paradox within the modern context. On one hand, they symbolize a return to the roots of health practices that appreciate the complex interplay between nature and the human body; on the other, they can serve as breeding grounds for misinformation, especially when extrapolated beyond their historical context and efficacy. The notion that apricot seeds could cure cancer poses a significant deviation from the healthy skepticism traditionally espoused by ancient practitioners, whose wisdom rejected one-size-fits-all remedies.

It is important to glean insights into ancient remedies without romanticizing them or accepting them as infallible. While many traditions continue to boast remarkable successes, particularly in preventive healthcare and minor illness management, the leap from historical practice to modern endorsement requires thorough investigation through the lenses of empirical research and clinical studies.

Examining the practices of the past offers a rich tapestry from which contemporary health advocates can draw inspiration. The narrative of historical herbalism reflects human ingenuity and adaptability, showcasing that even as we tread into the era of precision medicine, remnants of ancient wisdom can guide us in safeguarding our health choices against the tides of misinformation. Accruing knowledge not only demonstrates how far we have come but also reinforces the importance of questioning health claims—past and present—to ensure an informed approach towards wellness.

Thus, as we traverse the waning role of ancient remedies in a society propelled by scientific inquiry, we find ourselves at a cross-roads where history and modernity converge. The enduring allure of natural cures, including the tales surrounding apricot seeds, implores us to critically appraise their relevance today. In our quest for understanding, let us honor the wisdom of past generations while embracing a more discerning, evidence-based mindset that prioritizes safety and efficacy in our health decisions.

2.2. Folk Medicine and Its Modern Legacy

The exploration of folk medicine offers a captivating glimpse into the rich tapestry of human health practices and their evolution over millennia. In many cultures, folk medicine has served as a bridge between the natural world and the quest for healing, often reflecting broader societal beliefs, traditions, and knowledge systems. The legacy of folk medicine is layered, nuanced, and intrinsically tied to cultural narratives, shaping perceptions of health and wellness even in modern contexts.

Folk medicine encompasses a vast array of practices that are often localized, relying on regional flora, fauna, and indigenous wisdom. The roots of these practices can be traced back to pre-modern societies that relied heavily on empirical observations passed down through generations. Herbal remedies, poultices, tinctures, and various physical manipulations emerged as go-to solutions for ailments that plagued communities, deeply embedding themselves into the fabric of cultural identity. From Native American healing traditions that invoke the sacredness of the earth to the intricate systems found in Ayurveda and Traditional Chinese Medicine, folk health practices celebrate a holistic view of well-being rather than merely addressing symptomatic concerns.

The modern legacy of folk medicine is a dual-edged sword, celebrated for its capacity to harness natural resources while simultaneously criticized for perpetuating myths, particularly in the absence of robust scientific validation. In many contemporary societies, particularly in the West, folk medicine has been romanticized and often idealized, presenting a stark contrast to evidence-based practices. This allure of natural cures invites individuals to explore alternative pathways to health, especially in an age where pharmaceutical solutions are often questioned for their side effects and ethical implications.

Within this dynamic, the narrative surrounding apricot seeds emerges as a poignant case of misinformation derived from folk traditions. The kernels of apricots, rich in amygdalin—often misattributed as vitamin B17—garnered attention as a purported cancer cure. Advocates of the apricot seed narrative have transformed it into a tale of hope, drawing upon a framework shaped by folk medicine's acceptance of natural remedies. Yet, this allure is juxtaposed against a backdrop of solid scientific evidence that categorically dismisses the seeds as effective cancer treatments, instead highlighting the significant risks associated with their consumption due to cyanide poisoning.

The romanticization of folk cures like apricot seeds often derives from deep-seated cultural beliefs around the healing power of nature. For many, there remains an intrinsic yearning for simpler solutions, where the complex world of modern medicine feels alienating and overwhelming. The idea that a simple seed could wield the power to heal embodies hope and agency, propelling individuals to gravitate toward these narratives even when faced with contrary evidence. This psychological draw fosters a fertile ground for misinformation to flourish, illustrating how narratives sourced in folk medicine can become ingrained within popular consciousness.

Critical evaluation of the modern implications of folk remedies necessitates a balanced approach that respects traditional wisdom while embracing rigorous scientific inquiry. Folk medicine offers insights into historical practices that valued preventative health and community wellness, yet it must also evolve within the context of modern research methodologies. The challenge lies in distinguishing culturally cherished beliefs from scientifically substantiated claims. This is especially important as misinformation about natural remedies can lead individuals to forgo conventional treatments, ultimately endangering their health.

As we navigate this intricate landscape, it is essential to recognize the importance of building bridges between traditional healing practices and contemporary medical science. Initiatives that champion integrative health approaches, combining conventional medicine with effective elements of folk healing, can open doors to wider health equity. By fostering dialogues between practitioners trained in modern medicine and those knowledgeable in traditional healing methods, we can cultivate a richer understanding of health that respects diverse cultural practices while grounding treatment recommendations in scientific evidence.

The legacy of folk medicine is not merely a remnant of the past; it is an active, dynamic narrative that continues to shape health beliefs and practices today. Embracing this legacy means engaging with communities to honor their history while equipping them with the knowledge required to discern between beneficial remedies and potentially harmful myths. Through education and shared experiences, we can empower individuals to wield informed choices about their health, allowing for a future where the strengths of folk medicine enhance, rather than undermine, the advancements of modern science.

In conclusion, folk medicine's modern legacy propels critical conversations around health, healing, and cultural identity. As we unpack the intricate stories behind remedies like apricot seeds, we inevitably confront the challenges of misinformation and the ethical responsibilities we bear in promoting health. By valuing our ancestral wisdom while adhering to empirical evidence, we can navigate this historical continuum with clarity, ensuring that our health choices stem from a place of understanding rather than myth. As we look ahead, the pathway to wellness must bridge the past with the promise of advancements in science, creating a comprehensive approach to health that honors both tradition and innovation.

2.3. The Romanticism of Cure-All Remedies

The allure of cure-all remedies represents a captivating yet fraught perspective on health that has transcended centuries and cultures. This notion thrives on the desire for simplicity in healthcare, promising quick solutions to complex ailments, while fostering a romanticized vision of nature as the ultimate healer. During an era characterized by rapid advancements in technology and science, this desire remains a potent influence on public health beliefs, creating both opportunities and challenges in navigating medical truths versus myths.

At the heart of this phenomenon is the historical context in which natural remedies rose to prominence. Ancient civilizations, often lacking the empirical knowledge underpinning modern medicine, relied heavily on the resources available in their environments. Natural remedies were part of everyday life—cultivated through trial and error, strengthened by oral traditions, and steeped in cultural significance. These practices provided a sense of control and agency over health, igniting hope in communities that faced limited access to formal medical care. The pervasive narrative of nature's healing properties spurred the creation of countless herbal concoctions and remedies, fostering a belief in the power of a singular, simple solution to complex health issues.

The versatility and ease of natural remedies played a pivotal role in their romanticization. The idea that a single herb, root, or seed could offer miraculous benefits is inherently appealing. Consumers, especially those grappling with chronic ailments or serious diseases such as cancer, often yearn for straightforward solutions amidst torrent narratives of hopelessness. The apricot seed narrative epitomizes this desire; its proponents present the seed as possessing almost magical properties, capable of curing a disease dreaded by many. This characterization elevates the mundane apricot seed into an emblem of hope, reinforcing the notion that nature can triumph in the face of adversity.

the romanticization of cure-alls is not without consequences. As societal beliefs in these natural solutions grow, so does the potential for the spread of misinformation. The vital connection between anecdotal evidence and empirical research becomes blurred, leading individuals to make health decisions based on passion rather than scientific inquiry. The narrative of apricot seeds as a cancer cure stands as a testament to this dynamic: benign natural products are celebrated while their associated risks—namely, the toxicity of compounds like cyanide—remain conveniently sidelined. This selective narrative can inadvertently place lives at risk, a reality that sheds light on the darker side of hope promoted through romanticism.

Moreover, cultural factors hugely contribute to the persistence of these myths. Cross-generational knowledge transfer often means that folk beliefs become entrenched in collective consciousness, making it challenging to decipher where evidence ends and ideology begins. The appeal of the "natural" transcends scientific critique; it speaks to underlying values of self-reliance, simplicity, and a deep-seated mistrust of institutional authority. The effectiveness of pharmacological interventions and complex medical solutions may be overshadowed by the appealing simplicity offered by natural remedies, leading to a preference for unproven options.

Navigating through this romanticism necessitates a nuanced understanding of the interplay between belief and evidence. It encourages individuals to critically evaluate health claims and to seek a harmonious balance between ancient wisdom and modern science. The romantic allure of nature-based solutions is indeed compelling, but it should not overshadow the commitment to thorough research and scrutiny that modern medicine demands.

Critical engagement with the romanticism of cure-alls also dovetails into the discussions of informed health choices. Education plays an essential role in empowering consumers to make choices grounded in credible evidence rather than alluring narratives. By fostering health literacy, individuals are more equipped to discern potential risks from the genuine benefits of natural remedies. This balance does not imply a wholesale rejection of traditional practices; rather, it calls for an integrated approach that respects historical healing methods while ensuring rigorous validation through scientific exploration.

In conclusion, the romanticism of cure-all remedies, particularly in the context of apricot seeds, illustrates a complex relationship between hope, misinformation, and health. The allure of natural solutions must be tempered with informed decision-making based on empirical evidence and rigorous scrutiny. By embracing a well-rounded perspective that appreciates both traditional wisdom and modern science, we can pave the way for a healthcare landscape that honors diverse healing practices while prioritizing safety and effectiveness. As we navigate a world filled with health information, the challenge lies in distilling truth from myth, thereby fostering a future where informed choices lead to true wellness.

2.4. From Herbalism to Homeopathy

The narrative around herbalism, which finds its roots deep in ancient practices of healing, has always occupied a prestigious place in the pantheon of health. Essentially, herbalism embodies the systematic use of plants for medicinal purposes, built upon centuries of observation that revealed the potential of botanicals to alleviate suffering and restore health. This ancient practice flourished as communities recognized various plants' capacities to treat ailments, leading to their incorporation into both cultural and medicinal traditions. However, from its longstanding foundation, herbalism has evolved, intertwining with various other systems of thought and practice over the ages.

Track the developments through history, and you will observe the transition from simple herbal remedies to more complex systems of healing, including homeopathy. Homeopathy emerged in the late 18th century as a distinct philosophy rooted in the principles of "like cures like" and the law of infinitesimals – the idea that diluting a substance enhances its healing properties. Samuel Hahnemann, the founder of homeopathy, posited that a substance that causes symptoms in a healthy person could be used to treat similar symptoms in a sick person, a premise that marked a significant departure from the empirical practices of herbalism. While herbalism remains focused on employing specific plants or combinations for health benefits, homeopathy lifted this concept into a different realm of theoretical practice, emphasizing the dynamics of response and subtle energy shifts within the body.

At first, the allure of homeopathy bore resemblance to the appeal of herbal remedies—both offered a sense of hope and agency amid complex health landscapes often marred by uncertainty and fear. The 19th century was characterized by an increasing disillusionment with traditional medical practices, alongside calls for reform in how diseases were treated. Homeopathy, with its promise of safe, non-toxic remedies, quickly garnered fame and adherents. It captivated those seeking alternatives to the more invasive, and at times dangerous, treatments prescribed by conventional medicine, such as bloodletting and mercurial compounds.

However, as the lines between these modalities began to blur, the space between herbalism and homeopathy created an intriguing dichotomy that manifested in public consciousness. Many individuals, including some practitioners, became entangled in a curated narrative that suggested all that is natural is inherently good, thereby casting doubts on pharmaceutical treatments. This narrative, while appealing, has rendered consumers vulnerable to misinformation, fuelling the rise of unverified practices and products that lack rigorous scientific backing.

As we explore the particular case of apricot seeds in the context of both herbalism and homeopathy, we find ourselves at the nexus of belief and evidence—a fertile ground for myths about natural cures to flourish unchallenged. The seeds of apricots, rich in amygdalin, have been romanticized through various narratives as a powerful aid against cancer. Unfortunately, neither the herbalist paradigm nor the tenets of homeopathy can substantiate such claims with scientific rigor. While practitioners of herbalism may invoke the historical use of apricot seeds in traditional contexts, proponents of homeopathy lean into the rhetoric of energetic healing. Yet, both positions ultimately falter against the weight of contemporary research high-lighting the dangers associated with apricot seed consumption.

This brings us to a critical understanding: the distinction between these two approaches can often become nebulous, especially in popular discourse. Herbalism, with its strong emphasis on the therapeutic properties of specific plants, can blend seamlessly into the encapsulating philosophy of homeopathy, which seeks to find a more universal, subtle connection to healing. The problem arises when the safety of such remedies is taken for granted, and their perceived harmlessness leads individuals to overlook potential risks, both for themselves and others.

Concurrently, the movement toward integrative medicine—an increasingly popular approach that merges traditional healing systems with evidence-based practices—challenges both herbalist and homeopathic perspectives. Efforts to bridge the gap between these two philosophies have begun to lead towards a more cohesive understanding of health, acknowledging diverse modalities while advocating for critical evaluation of practices through scientific lenses.

In the case of apricot seeds, advocates intent on validating their supposed cancer-fighting capabilities may borrow elements from both herbalism and homeopathy—a careful selection of historical narratives and alternative healing principles—ultimately distorting their message. The seeds are framed as a simple, natural solution, echoing the long-standing paradigms of herbal cures, while simultaneously leveraging the trust in homeopathic principles by promoting the idea that their energy can heal the body at a fundamental level. Here lies the crux of the issue: while herbalism and homeopathy offer potential benefits, uncritical acceptance of the narratives attributed to apricot seeds can lead individuals down an unverified path with potentially grievous consequences.

To navigate this complexity requires critical discernment. As we cultivate our understanding of health practices, we must remain anchored in scrutiny and inquiry, ensuring that our beliefs about herbalism and homeopathy harmonize with scientifically validated outcomes. Persons seeking natural remedies should unearth the evidence surrounding these treatments, distinguishing between folklore and factual efficacy. By doing so, individuals uphold a commitment to informed health choices while fostering an environment where natural remedies can coexist with scientific inquiry, supporting holistic approaches that ultimately champion patient safety and well-being.

In conclusion, the journey from herbalism to homeopathy reveals a nuanced interplay between tradition, innovation, and critical inquiry in the realm of health. As narratives like those surrounding apricot seeds persist, it is our responsibility as health advocates and consumers to uphold standards of truth, ensuring that the paths we tread toward wellness remain illuminated by rigorous exploration and a commitment to safety. The rich tapestry woven from the threads of ancient wisdom and modern science continues to evolve, and the onus is upon us to navigate it thoughtfully, dedicated to what truly matters —our health and well-being.

2.5. Bridging Ancient Wisdom with Modern Science

The interplay between ancient wisdom and modern science creates a compelling narrative in the quest for health and healing. As we delve into this realm, we encounter the profound legacy of traditional practices that have stood the test of time, offering valuable insights into humanity's enduring relationship with nature and its resources. Ancient cultures possessed a remarkable understanding of their environmental surroundings, developing holistic approaches to health that embraced plants, minerals, and other natural substances for healing various ailments. This legacy, rife with the wisdom of generations, can serve as a foundation upon which modern scientific inquiry can build, ensuring that we do not lose sight of the enduring lessons of our ancestors.

In many societies, traditional medicine has been handed down through oral traditions and practical application, leading to the establishment of extensive knowledge systems that recognized the intricate connections between body, mind, and environment. For instance, Indigenous practices often emphasize the body's synergy with the natural world, advocating for a balance that promotes health and wellness. Similarly, traditional Chinese medicine and Ayurvedic practices highlight a comprehensive understanding of bodily systems and the importance of maintaining harmony for optimal health.

However, the advent of modern science has revolutionized our approach to health and healing, introducing rigorous methodologies that allow for the systematic study of disease, treatment, and overall health outcomes. The scientific method offers tools to discern truth from myth, guiding healthcare practices towards evidence-based solutions. While the cherished wisdom of the past remains valuable, it must coexist with empirical scrutiny to ensure that health recommendations prioritize safety and efficacy.

In bridging ancient wisdom with modern science, it is essential to adopt an integrative approach that respects the validity of traditional knowledge while adhering to the principles of scientific validation. This can be seen in eco-pharmacology, a growing field that examines the relationship between the environment, plant compounds, and human health. Researchers are forging new pathways by investigating the efficacy of traditional remedies through clinical trials and biomolecular studies, unearthing compounds that have shown therapeutic promise. This synthesis not only honors the knowledge of past generations but also breathes new life into their teachings, aligning them with contemporary scientific understanding.

A key aspect of this endeavor lies in the open-minded exchange of ideas between cultural practitioners and scientific researchers. Collaborative studies can yield rich rewards—an example being the examination of traditional herbal medicine from various cultures to inform modern pharmaceutical development. The exploration of compounds found in traditional treatments can lead to significant discoveries; for instance, many modern drugs have been derived from plants that were historically used to treat specific ailments. The resilence of these remedies across generations points to their potential effectiveness, a legacy that modern science is increasingly eager to validate.

However, the transition from ancient practices to contemporary medicine is not without challenges. Misinformation can arise easily when traditional practices are oversimplified or misrepresented in the context of modern health crises. The romantic allure of natural remedies can sometimes overshadow scientific understanding, leading consumers to embrace the narrative of 'nature as panacea' without deeming empirical evidence. The case of apricot seeds is an illustrative example of such misinformation: while they may have historical significance in traditional healing practices, their purported effectiveness against cancer is not substantiated and poses significant health risks.

Thus, as we draw the connections between ancient wisdom and modern science, it is vital that we remain vigilant against conflating these paradigms. This requires a disciplined approach to health information; stakeholders—be they practitioners, consumers, or educators —should critically assess health claims rooted in traditional practices. Open channels of communication between ancient wisdom advocates and modern scientists can bolster this narrative, ensuring that both parties learn from each other while prioritizing public safety.

The evolution of health communication in the digital age underscores the significance of navigating between these two realms effectively. The internet has become a multifaceted platform for information sharing, facilitating the exchange of knowledge between individuals seeking alternative health solutions rooted in tradition and scientific communities promoting evidence-based practices. However, the challenge lies in curating reliable sources and filtering misinformation, making health literacy a requirement in today's world. Consumers are increasingly empowered to seek information, yet they must also be equipped with the skills to discern legitimate health claims from dubious ones.

Bridging ancient wisdom with modern science ultimately serves as an invitation for ongoing dialogue—a discourse that opens pathways to integrating the strengths of both paradigms. By valuing the insights gleaned from traditional practices while applying the rigors of scientific inquiry, we can forge a path towards holistic health that honors the rich tapestry of human history while addressing the needs of modern society. This approach fosters an appreciation of our ancestral roots while aspiring to breakthroughs in contemporary healthcare, ensuring that wellness is both informed by the past and propelled by the future.

As we advance, let us remember that health choices are not merely a matter of following trends but rather an informed journey grounded in knowledge and understanding. The quest for wellness need not pose a dilemma between natural and conventional approaches; instead, it can become an integrated exploration, where ancient wisdom informs scientific progress, and modern science illuminates the richness of historical practices, enriching our disposition toward lifelong health.

3. The Rise and Appeal of Alternative Medicine

3.1. Understanding the Movement

As we explore the movement surrounding alternative medicine, it is essential to comprehend the underlying factors that have propelled its rise in popularity, specifically the interplay between skepticism towards conventional medicine and the appealing narratives touted by alternative practices. Understanding this movement requires an examination of historical context, cultural shifts, psychological influences, and contemporary challenges.

The roots of alternative medicine trace back to a growing discontent with conventional practices, particularly following events marked by public health crises and scandals involving pharmaceutical companies. Individuals began to question the motives behind traditional treatments and look for solutions that not only offered healing but also resonated with their cultural and philosophical beliefs regarding health and wellness. In this landscape, natural remedies emerged as proponents of a gentler, more holistic approach—contrasting sharply with the often invasive and aggressive nature of conventional medical treatments.

Fundamental to the allure of alternative medicine is the idea of empowerment. Many individuals find solace in the belief that they can exert control over their health decisions by opting for natural remedies. This sense of agency is often particularly appealing to those grappling with chronic illnesses, where conventional options may seem limited or fraught with side effects. Alternative medicine frameworks often provide narratives that emphasize self-determination, health sovereignty, and the body's innate ability to heal. Such rhetoric creates an environment of trust in natural pathways toward wellness and fosters a community of believers who value personal experience over empirical science.

Psychological dispositions also play a vital role in understanding the movement. Cognitive biases drive individuals towards information that validates their pre-existing beliefs, leading to confirmation bias. This phenomenon can significantly influence health-related decisions, as individuals gravitate toward alternative practices that align with their worldviews. Furthermore, the psychological comfort derived from natural therapies fills a vital emotional gap, often providing a sense of hope and connection, especially in times of despair associated with serious health conditions.

The narratives surrounding alternative treatments often encapsulate the simplicity and perceived safety of natural products. This simplicity, however, belies a complex reality; the inherent risks and potential dangers of these treatments are frequently downplayed. As exemplified in the case of apricot seeds, the promise of a simple, natural solution as a potential cancer cure enthralls many, despite mounting evidence of toxicity associated with their consumption. The romanticism of natural cures, bolstered by anecdotal testimonies, can easily overshadow sound scientific evidence, further complicating the landscape for potential patients.

The rise of the internet has dramatically influenced the alternative medicine movement. Access to information has grown exponentially, allowing individuals to explore health alternatives in unprecedented ways. Online platforms have enabled communities to form around shared experiences, while social media amplifies the narratives of natural healing, often turning personal testimonials into persuasive marketing tools. Sadly, however, the ease of disseminating information has also led to the proliferation of misinformation. The challenge lies in discerning credible sources from dubious claims—an increasingly difficult task for consumers navigating the complex web of online health advice.

This digital revolution has not only affected the accessibility of information but also shaped how individuals engage with health concerns. The immediacy of social media means that trends can go viral within a matter of hours, influencing public discourse and driving individuals towards unproven remedies. This can often occur incidentally, as individuals seeking community and support share their experiences without necessarily vetting the validity of their claims. The ensuing echo chambers breed a fertile ground for alternative medicine, where misinformation flourishes and substantiated science struggles to break through.

Importantly, the marketing of alternative medicine has evolved into a sophisticated industry that capitalizes on the appealing narrative of natural remedies while often masking scientific scrutiny. Companies selling products like apricot seeds can frame their offerings as harmless health enhancements, deftly sidestepping the negative implications of their use. In a world where the demand for natural cures persists, the line between, legitimate products and those not backed by sufficient evidence blurs alarmingly, confusing consumers further.

To navigate this landscape of alternative medicine requires critical thinking and a balanced perspective. As individuals seek to empower their health choices, it is vital to engage with evidence-based practices and expert opinions. One important step in enhancing this understanding is to cultivate health literacy, instilling an awareness of how to evaluate claims about remedies—natural or otherwise. This means identifying credible sources, asking pertinent questions, and seeking second opinions when faced with significant health decisions.

As we analyze the movement surrounding alternative medicine, it is also crucial to recognize that, while it is fueled by genuine desires for healing and improvement, it must be approached with caution. The appeal of alternative treatments cannot overshadow the importance of informed decision-making. Striking a balance between alternative and conventional practices—acknowledging each system's unique strengths and weaknesses—can lead to a more holistic and effective approach to health and wellness.

Ultimately, understanding the contemporary movement towards alternative medicine involves recognizing the underlying forces at play, the persuasive psychologies that guide health decisions, and the societal shifts contributing to this phenomenon. As we address the myriad challenges posed by misinformation, the distrust of conventional practices, and the intricate narratives surrounding natural remedies, we can foster dialogue that prioritizes safety, efficacy, and responsible healthcare choices for individuals seeking pathways to wellness.

3.2. The Influence of the Internet

The transformative role of the internet has created unprecedented opportunities and challenges in the realm of health information and decision-making. With its expansive reach, the internet remains a powerful platform for disseminating health-related knowledge, engaging individuals, and influencing health beliefs. However, with the myriad of information available, the veracity of claims can become clouded, leading to the propagation of myths and misinformation—especially in the context of alternative medicine and natural remedies like apricot seeds.

At the heart of this discussion lies the fact that the internet serves as both a blessing and a curse. On one hand, it democratizes access to information, enabling individuals to learn about health options, alternative therapies, and wellness trends at an unprecedented scale. This newfound access empowers individuals to seek out personalized healthcare solutions, fostering a sense of agency in an otherwise overwhelming medical landscape. The notion of self-directed health, supported by internet research, resonates particularly with individuals disillusioned by conventional treatments—those who feel overlooked, under-treated, or skeptical of pharmaceutical interventions.

In this digital age, websites, blogs, forums, and social media platforms allow people to share experiences and testimonials, creating a rich tapestry of collective narratives surrounding alternative treatments. The stories of individuals who have successfully turned to apricot seeds, or other natural remedies, for healing can rapidly circulate through social networks, captivating audiences with compelling anecdotes that sometimes overshadow scientific evidence. These testimonials, often laden with emotional weight, play a crucial role in shaping public perceptions, framing alternative remedies as viable solutions despite the lack of empirical support.

The ease with which information is shared online can contribute to the phenomenon of confirmation bias, where individuals selectively search for and interpret information that reinforces their preexisting beliefs. This mentality is particularly prevalent in health discussions, where users engage with content affirming their desire for natural cures, often dismissing or discrediting scientific perspectives. For instance, individuals who believe passionately in the cancer-fighting potential of apricot seeds may seek out anecdotal evidence or fringe studies that validate their convictions while ignoring extensive research that debunk these claims.

Moreover, social media platforms further amplify the influence of peer pressure and personal validation. The viral nature of social media can propel fringe health narratives to mainstream awareness, often disregarding context or the intricacies involved in scientific discourse. The overpowering presence of hashtags, viral posts, and trending challenges can create echo chambers, where misinformation breeds unquestioningly within supportive communities. In such environments, followers may feel social obligation to promote unverified health practices, isolating dissenting voices advocating for critical examination, and eroding trust in qualified healthcare professionals.

The spread of misinformation through the internet is compounded by the deliberate marketing of alternative remedies. Many businesses, selling apricot seeds and other unverified treatments, exploit the internet's reach to advertise products under the guise of authentic testimonials and natural advocacy. The marketing strategies employed often downplay the risks associated with these products in favor of persuasive narratives that equate natural with safe. This appeals to those seeking simple solutions to complex health issues, playing on fears and desires while neglecting critical discussions surrounding safety and efficacy.

In the face of this overwhelming tide of information, navigating health claims necessitates a critical lens. As consumers become increasingly tech-savvy and accustomed to seeking answers online, health literacy emerges as an essential skill. Individuals must be equipped with the tools to discern credible information from unreliable sources—a task that can be daunting given the sheer volume of content available. Educational initiatives designed to enhance health literacy can play a pivotal role in helping people identify scientific consensus and navigate the complexities of health information effectively.

Furthermore, the responsibility to combat misinformation does not lie solely with the consumer. Healthcare professionals and advocates must engage with digital spaces, providing clear, evidence-based information that counters misleading narratives. They can leverage the internet to promote accuracy, challenge myths, and share knowledge through various platforms that resonate with a diverse audience. This requires collaboration among researchers, healthcare practitioners, and tech experts to ensure that reliable data is not only accessible but presented in an engaging, user-friendly manner.

Ethical considerations also come into play, as there exists a moral imperative for influencers and health advocates to promote responsible health communication. Those who have significant platforms bear an obligation to fact-check information, acknowledge risks, and avoid sensationalizing treatments that may mislead their audience. Balancing the urge to share personal experiences with a commitment to accurate representation is vital in safeguarding public health.

Ultimately, the internet's influence on health beliefs underscores the need for a nuanced approach in our digital engagement. As we venture further into an era marked by rapid technological advancements, programmatic efforts must also reflect an understanding of the complexities of human psychology, cultural beliefs, and the narratives surrounding health. Promoting informed health choices requires a collaborative effort to reconcile historical wisdom, personal experience, and the rigor of scientific inquiry—and the internet can serve as the bridge that connects these diverse elements.

As we continue to explore the nuances of health information online, we must prioritize clarity, evidence, and empathy in our communication. Fostering constructive dialogues around health issues will enable individuals to make informed choices that ultimately benefit their well-being, steering them away from the perils of misinformation and toward pathways of genuine health advocacy and empowerment. In navigating this sprawling landscape, we must remain vigilant, promoting a culture of questioning and validating claims, while fostering an understanding of health that is grounded in both ancient wisdom and modern science.

3.3. Case Studies of Alternative Success Stories

In illuminating the landscape of alternative medicine, the narratives surrounding successful outcomes and personal testimonials are compelling tools that amplify the idea of natural remedies. These case studies often provide an emotionally rich context that captivates audiences and fosters a sense of community around shared experiences. While it is vital to approach these anecdotes with critical scrutiny, they also offer valuable insights into the complexities of healing practices, showcasing instances where patients have reported positive outcomes from alternative approaches—or the persuasive narratives surrounding them.

One crucial case study involves a group of patients seeking relief from chronic illnesses, including cancer, through the exploration of alternative therapies. These individuals often form support networks that emphasize their shared commitment to holistic health and natural remedies. Testimonials emerge from these communities, glorifying the healing properties of substances like apricot seeds, which are often celebrated as part of an integrative lifestyle. Such personal accounts can garner powerful emotional resonance, transforming individual experiences into a collective movement advocating for natural solutions. Individuals frequently cite improved well-being and a sense of empowerment, nurturing a belief that they can take control of their healing journey. Yet, the narrative of success in these scenarios can overshadow the complexity of each case, leading to an incomplete understanding of the potential outcomes—both beneficial and adverse.

In a notable instance documented in wellness blogs and social media, a patient with stage IV cancer opted to include apricot seed consumption as part of her alternative therapy protocol. Over several months, she reported subjective improvements in her quality of life, attributing these changes to the seeds and an array of dietary changes that she had implemented. Her story, filled with positivity and hope, became a rallying point for many others searching for non-traditional healing. The compelling nature of her account was further buoyed by a robust online presence, where her journey was actively shared and discussed. Here lies an example of how testimonial narratives can inadvertently foster a belief in efficacy, even when rigorous scientific evidence fails to support such claims.

However, it is crucial to note that these accounts often lack the scientific rigor needed to validate the effectiveness of the treatments being espoused. Variables such as placebo effects, dietary changes, psychological resilience, and standard medical treatments can contribute to positive outcomes in ways that anecdotal evidence cannot isolate or evaluate. In the case of the aforementioned patient, there is a cautionary note in that her subjective improvements may not directly correlate to the consumption of apricot seeds, but rather the result of multiple factors—each individually taking part in her holistic journey toward health.

A contrasting case study can be found in a cohort of patients who suffered adverse effects from the unregulated consumption of apricot seeds. While some users report positive experiences without immediate consequences, others have faced dire health repercussions due to cyanide poisoning, which is linked to amygdalin—a compound found in the seeds. As a result, the stark reality emerges that while some may proclaim triumphs, others may suffer devastating health crises. This raises fundamental ethical concerns about the promotion of alternative treatments lacking robust regulation or accountability.

Similarly, integrating the experiences of patients who have benefitted from established alternative treatments—such as acupuncture, herbal therapies, or dietary interventions—can provide a more nuanced understanding of alternative medicine's capacity to complement conventional approaches. In these instances, the integration of practices rooted in both traditional knowledge and modern understanding can lead to positive health outcomes. For example, cases involving patients undergoing cancer treatment alongside acupuncture therapy often report reduced side effects and enhanced well-being. Such integrative approaches highlight the potential for evidence-based alternatives that harness the strengths of various methodologies while upholding patient safety.

Examining these varied narratives reveals a paradox: while some patients find solace and success in alternative practices, others may encounter risk and misinformation. Bridging this divide requires a commitment to critical examination and a cautious approach to claims. It is vital to engage with communities not only to explore their experiences but also to guide them toward reliable information and practices supported by evidence.

Moreover, the wider implications of these case studies extend to healthcare policies and public awareness campaigns aimed at mitigating misinformation regarding alternative medicine. By synthesizing individual experiences with evidence-based guidance, we can contribute to the global discourse on health decision-making and patient autonomy.

In summary, the case studies of alternative success stories illustrate a complex interplay between individual narratives, community engagement, and health outcomes. While the emotional allure of personal testimonies can be powerful in shaping the perception of treatments like apricot seeds, there is an imperative need for rigorous scientific validation to support or refute these claims. As healthcare advocates, we must foster informed dialogue that emphasizes the importance of considering both anecdotal evidence and scientific inquiry, ensuring a balanced approach to health choices within the ever-evolving landscape of alternative medicine.

3.4. The Role of Peer Influence

The capacity for peer influence in health choices, especially regarding alternative medicine, is a factor of immense significance that warrants a comprehensive exploration. In an age where information is abundant yet often conflicting, the sway of peers can shape beliefs and decisions in profound ways. This form of influence draws upon a mix of psychological, social, and cultural dimensions, intricately woven together through personal experiences, social validation, and the desire for acceptance within communities.

Within any social group, individuals naturally seek connections with others who share similar beliefs and values. This fundamental aspect of human interaction is amplified in health discussions, where the complexity and emotional weight of health-related decisions can be overwhelming. Individuals often turn to their peers for guidance, feedback, and affirmation—especially in matters that involve significant risks or fears. The narratives surrounding natural remedies like apricot seeds often gain traction not only through scientific backing but also through personal anecdotes shared within social circles. These anecdotes provide social proof, fostering a sense of belonging as individuals resonate with experiences that echo their own health concerns or aspirations.

The rise of social media has elevated the role of peer influence to unprecedented levels. Platforms like Facebook, Instagram, and TikTok create environments where people readily share their health journeys and decisions, allowing personal stories to reach wider audiences. A single viral post about the benefits of apricot seeds, supported by emotive testimonials and engaging visuals, can lead many to adopt these practices without a thorough consideration of the accompanying risks. When peers celebrate these narratives, the psychological impact can be substantial. Individuals may feel an implicit obligation to align with the trending health views promoted by friends or influencers, often prioritizing communal endorsement over critical evaluation or scientific reasoning.

Moreover, peer influence often intersects with cognitive biases, particularly confirmation bias, wherein individuals gravitate towards information that validates their pre-existing beliefs. When a small group of friends collectively espouses the belief in the cancer-fighting properties of apricot seeds, it becomes increasingly challenging for dissenting opinions to penetrate that echo chamber. The communal reinforcement of these ideas can lead to a shared conviction that overrides skepticism or caution, pushing individuals toward decisions that might not be in their best interest.

The narrative surrounding apricot seeds serves as a poignant example of these dynamics at play. Individuals who have witnessed a loved one adopt apricot seeds into their cancer regimen may recount their experience with dramatic flair, emphasizing remarkable "recoveries" or improvements. This can inadvertently create a powerful incentive for others to try the seeds themselves, disregarding crucial information about the potential dangers, such as cyanide toxicity, associated with consumption. In this instance, peer influence operates on an emotional level, invoking hope and a sense of empowerment for those seeking alternatives to conventional medicine.

Cultural contexts also magnify the impact of peer influence on health decisions. In communities that prioritize traditional healing or alternative medicine, narratives championing natural remedies can become deeply entrenched within cultural identities. When these remedies are celebrated at community gatherings or disseminated through traditional communication channels, they gain an elevated status that legitimizes their use. Conversely, any critical stance on these remedies may be met with resistance, as it threatens to disrupt the communal fabric woven around these shared beliefs.

Understanding the role of peer influence is paramount for public health advocacy and education. As misinformation and myths about remedies like apricot seeds proliferate, it becomes critical to foster discussions that enable individuals to challenge group norms responsibly. This involves promoting health literacy, encouraging critical thinking, and enabling individuals to seek out reliable sources of information. One strategy could be to create environments that foster open dialogue about diverse health practices, inviting questions and dissent rather than simply reinforcing existing narratives.

Innovative approaches tailored to counteract the influence of unreliable peer information can facilitate a more balanced discourse. Health campaigns that utilize testimonials from trusted healthcare professionals can provide a counter-narrative to the stories proliferating through social circles. By leveraging the credibility of medical experts alongside community engagement initiatives, public health messaging can reach individuals when they are most susceptible to peer influence, injecting verified scientific information into conversations typically dominated by anecdotal evidence.

In conclusion, the role of peer influence in health decision-making is a multifaceted phenomenon that stems from intrinsic human connections, social dynamics, and cultural narratives. Recognizing the complexity of this influence is necessary in addressing the health myths and misinformation surrounding unproven remedies like apricot seeds. Public health efforts that prioritize education, critical engagement, and the integration of diverse scientific perspectives into community discussions can foster more informed choices among individuals navigating these treacherous waters. In the quest for wellness, the capacity to leverage peer influence positively holds immense promise for guiding health decisions towards evidence-based practices, thereby reinforcing a collective commitment to factual accuracy and patient safety.

3.5. Navigating Between Conventional and Alternative Paths

As individuals navigate the complex terrain of health decisions, the decision-making process often finds itself caught in a delicate balance between conventional and alternative paths. The surge of interest in alternative medicine is not simply a reflection of personal choice, but rather a nuanced interplay of factors, including dissatisfaction with conventional treatments, cultural beliefs about natural remedies, and the pervasive influence of peer networks. For many, alternative medicine represents hope—the possibility of a more holistic, less invasive approach to health. This subchapter seeks to explore how individuals can wisely navigate between these often-conflicting health paradigms.

At the core of this navigation process is the need to foster an understanding of both conventional and alternative medicine. While conventional treatments are often grounded in rigorous scientific research and evidence-based practices, alternative therapies frequently draw from historical and cultural knowledge systems that have persisted for generations. Therein lies a challenge: how do individuals maintain an open mind to the potential benefits of alternative remedies without compromising their health by eschewing sound medical advice?

The journey begins with self-awareness. Patients must assess their own beliefs and feelings towards health and healing, reflecting on past experiences with healthcare professionals, treatments, and outcomes. This introspection can illuminate biases that may unduly influence decisions. For example, disillusionment with pharmaceutical companies—spurred by media reports of unethical practices—can lead individuals to gravitate towards natural remedies. Here, critical thinking plays a crucial role in separating valid concerns from unfounded fears, ensuring that health choices are informed rather than driven by anecdotal evidence or emotional appeals.

One useful framework for navigating these paths is the concept of integrative medicine. This approach seeks to bridge the gap between conventional and alternative therapies, emphasizing the strength of a patient-centered model that considers the patient's values, preferences, and unique health circumstances. Integrative medicine integrates assessments from multiple disciplines, allowing for a comprehensive understanding of the individual and their condition. This framework legitimizes the inclusion of alternative treatments—such as dietary supplements or mind-body techniques—while concurrently advocating for the continued reliance on scientifically validated medical practices. Patients could benefit from the collaborative efforts of medical doctors and practitioners of alternative therapies working side by side, fostering a dialogue that respects both traditions.

Furthermore, individuals must actively engage in research. Health literacy—the ability to access, comprehend, and evaluate health information—is essential in making informed choices. This means developing the skill to discern credible sources of information from those that perpetuate myths. Engaging with peer-reviewed journals, reputable health organizations, and verified resources can empower individuals to make choices based on facts rather than speculative claims. As examples abound regarding the hazards of unverified treatments—such as the notorious apricot seed narrative—awareness of supporting evidence becomes critical.

Community plays an equally important role in the navigation process. People often turn to their social circles for guidance, deeply influenced by the experiences and opinions of peers. While personal stories and testimonials can be compelling, they can also be deceptive. Visitors to alternative medicine forums, for instance, might encounter users praising the efficacy of treatments that lack scientific validation. In this light, it is vital for individuals to develop a discerning eye, questioning the underlying motivations, biases, and accuracy of such narratives. Open discussions within peer networks about health practices can lead to well-rounded perspectives, potentially steering individuals toward evidence-based conclusions.

The influence of social media cannot be overstated; it serves as both a beacon of information and a minefield of misinformation. Platforms like Instagram and Facebook facilitate the spread of health narratives, where personal stories of triumph in the fight against illness often overshadow scientific discourse. As individuals seek solutions to their health challenges, they must remain vigilant against the allure of sensational claims and consider the broader context before making any decisions. Joining supportive groups where balanced discussions take place can help counteract the potential negative impacts of echo chambers that reinforce misleading or harmful views, particularly surrounding unregulated treatments.

When exploring alternative remedies, it is also crucial to engage healthcare professionals in a collaborative dialogue. Patients should not hesitate to discuss their interests in complementary therapies with their medical providers. These conversations can foster mutual respect and understanding. A practitioner knowledgeable about both conventional and alternative methods may guide patients toward safe and effective integration, enabling them to explore their interests while ensuring their primary health needs remain a priority.

The importance of informed consent cannot be overstated when making choices about treatments. Individuals should not only be aware of what they are opting to pursue but must also consider the potential risks associated with alternative options. Empirical evidence surrounding the use of natural remedies—such as apricot seeds— demands scrutiny, given its potential to mislead patients despite its allure. Individuals must remain informed about existing research and any established warnings regarding unproven remedies and engage in discussions with healthcare providers about their validity.

For those considering alternative medicine, balancing the promise of natural solutions with the proven efficacy of conventional medical treatments can provide a well-rounded approach to health. Embracing an open and collaborative spirit while prioritizing evidence-based practices enables individuals to navigate this intricate landscape with confidence and awareness.

Navigating between conventional and alternative paths presents a multifaceted challenge, fueled by a confluence of emotions, experiences, beliefs, and relationships. By cultivating critical thinking, engaging with accurate resources, fostering discussions with healthcare professionals, and valuing community relationships built on transparency and respect, individuals can make empowered health choices. In such a dynamic environment, the ongoing dialogue between alternative and conventional medicine must continue, with the overarching goal of promoting safe, informed, and effective care tailored to the needs of each individual. Ultimately, the journey toward optimal health is about finding the right balance—one that recognizes the value in both tradition and innovation, paving the way for a more holistic and enriched understanding of wellness.

4. The Science of Cancer: An Overview

4.1. Defining Cancer: A Malignant Evolution

Cancer is a term that encapsulates a spectrum of diseases character-ized by the uncontrolled growth and spread of abnormal cells within the body. This malignant evolution stems from various genetic, envi-ronmental, and lifestyle factors that transform normal cells into rogue agents capable of disregarding the biological rules governing growth and replication. Understanding cancer necessitates a closer look at its definition, the underlying biological mechanisms driving tumori-genesis, and its evolving nature.

At its core, cancer arises when there is a disturbance in the balance of cell division and cell death. The human body functions through a meticulously coordinated system of checks and balances that reg-ulates cellular processes. In a healthy state, cells are instructed to grow, divide, and die according to the synchronized signals from their environment. However, in cancerous cells, these regulatory pathways become destabilized due to mutations in critical genes—specifically those involved in cell cycle control, apoptosis (programmed cell death), and DNA repair mechanisms.

The defining feature of cancer is its heterogeneity; it is not a single disease but rather a complex group of over 100 different types, each with distinct characteristics, behaviors, and responses to treatment. The World Health Organization (WHO) classifies cancers based on the tissues where they originate, including carcinomas (epithelial cells), sarcomas (connective tissues), leukemias (hematopoietic cells), lymphomas (lymphatic system cells), and melanomas (melanocytes). Despite this classification system, the intricacies of cancer develop-ment transcend mere anatomical location, leading to a need for a more detailed understanding of tumor biology and behavior.

Mutations play a critical role in the evolution of cancer cells. These genetic alterations can occur through various mechanisms, ranging from copying errors during DNA replication to exposure to environ-mental carcinogens such as tobacco smoke, radiation, and certain chemicals. Mutations may be categorized into three primary types: oncogenes, tumor suppressor genes, and DNA repair genes. Oncogenes, when mutated, promote excessive cell division or survival, while tumor suppressor genes typically serve as "brakes" on cell proliferation, and their loss of function contributes to tumor growth. The failure of DNA repair genes results in the accumulation of mutations, further driving malignancy.

Beyond genetic mutations, cancer initiation and progression can also be significantly influenced by epigenetics, which involves changes in gene expression without altering the underlying DNA sequence. External factors, including diet, lifestyle, and environmental exposures, can lead to epigenetic modifications that in turn affect cancer development. Research indicates that alterations to the epigenome may play a role in a tumor's ability to metastasize, evade the immune system, and develop resistance to treatment.

The microenvironment surrounding a tumor further complicates cancer's biological framework. Interactions between cancer cells and surrounding normal cells, including immune cells, fibroblasts, and blood vessels, can facilitate tumor growth and promote metastasis—the process by which cancer spreads to other parts of the body. The tumor microenvironment can provide a support system that nourishes cancer cells, granting them the resources necessary to thrive. Importantly, it is within this interplay that the distinction between benign and malignant processes becomes stark; while benign tumors may grow locally without invading other tissues, malignant tumors possess the unique ability to breach tissue boundaries and establish secondary tumors, complicating treatment and decreasing survival probabilities.

As we look at the broader societal context, the rising prevalence of cancer underscores the need to address both prevention and treatment comprehensively. With the burden of disease expanding globally, awareness of modifiable risk factors—such as smoking cessation, physical activity, and diet—becomes paramount. Simultaneously, ongoing advancements in cancer research aim to unravel the intricacies of tumor biology, paving the way for personalized treatment approaches that target the specific molecular characteristics of a patient's cancer. The future of oncological care lies in the intersection of technology, biology, and human experience, with the promise of innovations in immunotherapy, targeted therapy, and early detection methods poised to enhance patient outcomes dramatically.

Understanding cancer as a malignant evolution reveals the complex interplay of genetic, environmental, and lifestyle factors that contribute to this multifaceted disease. This perspective invites a deeper inquiry into the transformative nature of cancer, challenging us to rethink historical narratives surrounding its origins and treatment, including the lure of natural remedies like apricot seeds. Ultimately, the pursuit of knowledge in the realm of cancer biology is vital, for it underscores the imperative to develop effective strategies for prevention, treatment, and improved outcomes for future generations.

4.2. Genetics, Mutations, and Risks

Genetics provides the fundamental blueprint of life, intricately woven into the complex tapestry of human health. In the context of cancer, understanding genetics is essential as it plays a pivotal role in cellular behavior, governing how mutations arise, proliferate, and ultimately shape the risk profiles of individuals. Recognizing the nuanced interplay of genetic factors lays the groundwork for comprehending the broader implications tied to cancer, particularly in dissecting the myths surrounding alternative treatments like apricot seeds.

At the molecular level, cancer originates from genetic mutations that disturb the normal regulatory functions within a cell. These mutations can occur in two primary types of genes: oncogenes and tumor suppressor genes. Oncogenes are mutated forms of normal genes (proto-oncogenes) that promote cell division or survival. In contrast, tumor suppressor genes typically act as guardians against unchecked growth by regulating the cell cycle and facilitating programmed cell death, or apoptosis. When these genes mutate, either through inherited conditions or external environmental factors such as radiation and carcinogens, the delicate balance between cellular proliferation and death is disrupted, fostering the uncontrolled cell growth characteristic of cancer.

One crucial aspect of genetic mutations is its dual nature: some mutations are benign, while others can have profound implications for individual health. The concept of genetic predisposition highlights how certain individuals may inherit mutations that significantly increase their cancer risk. For example, mutations in the BRCA1 and BRCA2 genes are notably linked to breast and ovarian cancers, prompting discussions around genetic screening for those with a family history of such ailments. Understanding one's genetic makeup can empower individuals to take proactive measures—such as increased surveillance or opting for preventive surgeries—to mitigate their risk effectively.

However, genetics alone does not narrate the entire story. Environmental factors intricately interact with genetic predispositions, giving rise to multifactorial conditions like cancer—where genetics, lifestyle choices, and environmental exposures converge. For instance, while an individual may carry a genetic mutation predisposing them to cancer, it is often the interplay with factors such as diet, tobacco use, physical activity, and exposure to toxic substances that may trigger the actual onset of the disease. This interplay complicates the cancer narrative, as individuals employ various avenues to navigate threats to their health, including gravitating towards natural remedies like apricot seeds, often believed to mitigate cancer risk.

The rise of alternative medicine, with its host of unverified remedies, echoes the complexities surrounding public perception of cancer risk. Individuals seeking solace from overwhelming fears of cancer often latch onto narratives that promise relief, embodying the hope for natural interventions. Within this context, the belief in apricot seeds as a cancer-fighting agent, hinged on their cyanogenic properties, takes center stage. Advocates of this narrative tout the presence of amygdalin, purportedly a form of vitamin B17, as imperative in thwarting cancer cell proliferation. However, it is critical to differentiate between anecdotal claims and scientific evidence, as the consumption of apricot seeds carries the potential for toxicity leading to cyanide poisoning.

Numerous studies have contextually laid bare the inherent risks associated with apricot seeds. While proponents may cite isolated cases of individuals claiming health improvements following the incorporation of apricot seeds into their regimen, these stories fail to acknowledge the significant instances of adverse reactions following their consumption. Notably, the very component that proponents champion—amygdalin—poses a danger when metabolized in the body, revealing the critical need to scrutinize both traditional beliefs and modern trends.

The scientific community overwhelmingly advocates for informed decision-making rooted in empirical evidence. The consensus is clear: while genetics provides insights into susceptibility and risk, it must be contextualized within a framework of rigorous scientific inquiry. This context extends to alternative treatments that promise solutions amid the complex landscape of cancer. Relying on unvalidated claims offers a false sense of security, leaving individuals vulnerable to misinformation and potentially detrimental health choices.

Genetics, mutations, and risks converge to shape the multifaceted narrative of cancer—a narrative that demands thoughtful exploration and critical understanding. Proponents of remedies like apricot seeds inadvertently traverse an intricate path between belief and empirical fact, driving conversations around health behaviors, informed decision-making, and the ethical implications of alternative medicine.

The journey through cancer prevention and treatment is informed by a tapestry of knowledge—the interplay between genetics and environmental exposures offers a rich understanding of the risks involved. Recognizing the power of the genetic narrative does not diminish the contributions of lifestyle and environmental factors that play integral roles in cancer development. Therefore, awareness and education become paramount in equipping individuals to engage with the landscape of health choices responsibly.

As we provoke conversations surrounding the narratives of cancer risk, including the alluring myths of apricot seeds, we must consistently advocate for informed health literacy. Balancing the allure of natural remedies with a commitment to scientific inquiry ensures that individuals navigate their health journeys empowered by knowledge and guided by evidence, ultimately fostering well-informed decisions that promote wellness in the long term. In a world filled with messages of hope, it is our duty to emphasize the importance of authenticity—a practice that prioritizes health, safety, and well-being.

4.3. Traditional Cancer Treatments Explained

Traditional cancer treatments encompass a range of approaches developed through decades of rigorous scientific research and clinical practice. These treatments form the backbone of modern oncology and have evolved significantly over time, integrating advances in medical technology and biochemistry. In this exploration, we will thoroughly examine the primary modalities used in cancer treatment, their mechanisms of action, and their implications for patients, juxtaposed against the narrative of alternative remedies, such as those surrounding apricot seeds.

Surgical intervention remains one of the oldest and most effective forms of cancer treatment. The primary intent of surgery is to physically remove tumors along with surrounding tissue, often aiming for the best possible margin of healthy cells to minimize recurrence. This treatment is most effective for localized cancers, those not yet spread beyond the original site. Surgical options can range from lumpectomies, where only a portion of the breast tissue is removed, to radical procedures such as mastectomies or the resection of entire organs affected by malignancies. The success of surgical treatment depends significantly on the timing of the procedure—early detection allows for better prognoses and, ultimately, improved survival rates.

Radiation therapy is another cornerstone of cancer treatment that employs high-energy particles or waves to destroy or incapacitate cancer cells. Two primary forms of radiation therapy exist: external beam radiation, which targets the tumor from outside the body, and brachytherapy, where radioactive material is implanted directly into or near the tumor. This modality primarily functions by damaging DNA within cancer cells, leading to cell death. While effective, radiation therapy can also affect nearby healthy tissue, resulting in side effects that range from fatigue to localized skin problems, depending on the treatment area. Advances in technology, such as Intensity-Modulated Radiation Therapy (IMRT) and Proton Therapy, continue to refine the accuracy and reduce collateral damage associated with radiation treatment.

Chemotherapy is a systemic cancer treatment that utilizes cytotoxic drugs to kill rapidly dividing cells, a hallmark of cancerous cells. Typically, chemotherapy regimens consist of a combination of drugs administered over a series of cycles to maximize effectiveness and minimize resistance. This treatment can be particularly effective for cancers that have metastasized, as well as those that are not amenable to surgery. However, the non-specific nature of these drugs means they can also harm normal, rapidly dividing cells, leading to a range of side effects such as nausea, hair loss, and fatigue. As research progresses, personalized chemotherapy regimens based on the genetic profile of the tumor aim to enhance efficacy and reduce adverse effects.

Targeted therapy represents a revolutionary evolution in oncology, focusing on specific molecular targets associated with cancer. By honing in on the unique characteristics of cancer cells—such as specific proteins or genetic mutations—these therapies can disrupt the interchange of signals that promote tumor growth. Agents like trastuzumab (Herceptin) for HER2-positive breast cancer or imatinib (Gleevec) for chronic myeloid leukemia exemplify the power of targeted therapies. While they have shown remarkable success in improving outcomes for certain patient populations, the complexity of cancer biology necessitates ongoing research to develop novel targets and treatments for a broader array of cancer types.

Immunotherapy is garnering significant attention as a new frontier in cancer treatment, relying on the body's immune system to recognize and destroy cancer cells. This includes treatments such as monoclonal antibodies, cancer vaccines, and immune checkpoint inhibitors, such as pembrolizumab (Keytruda) and nivolumab (Opdivo). These therapies aim to bolster the immune system's natural defenses, shifting the balance towards a more effective anti-tumor response. Like many therapies, immunotherapy can provoke immune-related side effects, necessitating careful monitoring and management.

Combination therapy, which integrates multiple treatment modalities, reflects the increasingly complex landscape of cancer treatment. A combination of surgery, radiation, chemotherapy, targeted therapies, and immunotherapies can optimize patient outcomes. The selection of a treatment plan is tailored to the individual patient, considering factors such as cancer type, stage, patient health status, and the presence of specific biomarkers.

Potential patients often face overwhelming choices in a climate celebrating natural remedies as effective alternatives. In the context of treatments like apricot seeds, narratives surrounding their supposed cancer-fighting properties can present significant challenges. It must be emphasized that these claims lack credible scientific substantiation and pose risks due to the seeds' potential toxicity, particularly concerning cyanide poisoning.

Confronting the narrative of alternative treatments alongside established modalities is vital for fostering informed health choices. As individuals seek solace in natural remedies amid searching for options that better resonate with their beliefs, it becomes crucial to advocate for evidence-based approaches and dissuade reliance on unproven treatments. While the allure of apricot seeds may captivate some, ignoring rigorous scientific evaluation and established treatments like chemotherapy, targeted therapy, and immunotherapy may risk delaying crucial interventions.

In summary, traditional cancer treatments—surgery, radiation, chemotherapy, targeted therapy, and immunotherapy—stand as testaments to innovation grounded in scientific research. While the efficacy and safety of these methods continue to evolve, their roles underscore the need for informed decision-making in cancer care. As we navigate the waters of alternative therapies, including those steeped in tradition and myth, ongoing engagement with credible evidence remains imperative in championing patient health and wellness. By prioritizing scientifically validated approaches, we not only empower individuals but also honor the complexity of cancer and the knowledge gleaned from years of dedicated research and clinical innovation.

4.4. Breakthroughs in Cancer Research

As we delve into the landscape of cancer research, we encounter a compelling and fast-moving domain where innovations, advancements, and groundbreaking discoveries unfold with remarkable frequency. The ceaseless pursuit for effective cancer treatments has spurred a series of breakthroughs that revolutionize the way we understand, diagnose, and treat this complex group of diseases. Each significant discovery not only enhances the scientific community's grasp of cancer biology but also reshapes clinical practices, empowering patients and providing new avenues of hope.

In recent years, the field of cancer research has made significant strides, intertwining modern technological innovations with classic biological inquiry. The Human Genome Project, completed in 2003, revolutionized the scientific approach to understanding cancer at the molecular level. By unveiling the complete genetic blueprint of humanity, researchers gleaned insights into the genetic variations and mutations that contribute to cancer development. This foundational knowledge laid the groundwork for precision medicine, enabling targeted therapies that tailor treatments to the specific genetic profile of each tumor.

Precision oncology stands out as one of the landmark advancements in cancer treatment. At its core, precision oncology seeks to personalize treatment regimens by assessing the unique genetic makeup of a patient's cancer cells. Tumors often harbor specific mutations that can be therapeutically targeted, allowing for drugs to directly attack dysfunctional pathways within cancer cells. For instance, the discovery of mutations in the EGFR gene led to the emergence of targeted therapies such as erlotinib, providing effective treatments for non-small cell lung cancer patients. The tailored approach marks a paradigm shift from traditional one-size-fits-all methods, aligning treatment strategies with the biological underpinnings of individual tumors.

Moreover, immunotherapy has emerged as a powerful player in the cancer research arena. By harnessing the body's own immune system to recognize and combat tumor cells, immunotherapy has shown remarkable promise across various cancer types. Immune checkpoint inhibitors, such as pembrolizumab and nivolumab, disrupt the pathways that tumors use to evade immune detection, ultimately reinvigorating the immune response against the malignancy. These therapies have transformed previously intractable cancers, such as melanoma and certain lymphomas, into manageable diseases. The potential of immunotherapy continues to stimulate research efforts as scientists work to refine these treatments and expand their applicability to other cancer types.

The integration of artificial intelligence (AI) and machine learning into cancer research represents another fascinating frontier. Researchers employ AI algorithms to mine vast datasets, identifying patterns, predicting outcomes, and optimizing treatment pathways. The extensive use of imaging technologies coupled with AI's analytical capabilities has the ability to revolutionize diagnostic practices. For instance, deep learning models are increasingly used to assess radiological images faster and more accurately than human experts, leading to earlier detection and improved prognoses. This technology is also applied to genomic data, enabling the identification of novel mutations and potential therapeutic targets.

Furthermore, the potential of liquid biopsies in the realm of early cancer detection has profound implications for the future of cancer diagnostics and patient management. Liquid biopsies analyze circulating tumor DNA (ctDNA) from blood samples, offering a non-invasive approach to detecting cancer and monitoring treatment responses. This innovation allows for continuous assessment of tumors, enabling healthcare providers to glean insights without the need for repetitive invasive procedures. The ability to track genetic changes and mutations over time in real-time stands to empower oncologists in adapting treatment strategies and enhancing patient survival outcomes.

On the horizon of cancer research, advancements in combinatorial therapy hold great promise. The interplay between different therapeutic modalities—whether it be combining immunotherapy with chemotherapy, radiation, or targeted treatments—can bolster therapeutic effectiveness and overcome resistance mechanisms that may render single-agent therapies ineffective. Researchers continuously explore synergistic relationships between drugs, pushing the boundaries of what treatment regimens can achieve in tackling complex malignancies.

The emergence of patient-centered research initiatives further emphasizes the necessity of including patient perspectives in the development of new interventions. Researchers recognize the importance of establishing collaborative partnerships with patients, seeking to understand the experience of those affected by cancer and how treatments impact their quality of life. This movement encapsulates the shift towards holistic care, ensuring that research not only focuses on clinical outcomes but also addresses the psychological and emotional needs of patients navigating their cancer journeys.

Despite the remarkable advancements achieved through interdisciplinary research efforts, challenges persist. The complexity of cancer biology, coupled with the heterogeneity of tumors across individuals, often complicates treatment outcomes, underscoring the need for ongoing inquiry and collaboration among scientists, clinicians, and patients. Navigating the intricacies of regulatory approvals for new therapies, managing costs, and ensuring equitable access to innovative treatments also demands attention.

As we reflect on the significant breakthroughs in cancer research, the landscape becomes clear: the combination of technological innovation, personalized medicine, and patient involvement has the potential to redefine the future of cancer treatment. In this age marked by collaboration and shared knowledge, the hope fostered by scientific discovery transcends traditional boundaries, offering a beacon of light for all those impacted by this complex disease.

Integrating these advancements into clinical practice necessitates a commitment to ongoing education, awareness, and advocacy in the health community. As we embrace the future of cancer research, it is vital to enhance public understanding of these developments and empower patients with the knowledge needed to navigate their health proactively. By aligning modern breakthroughs with ethical considerations and patient-centered approaches, we can pave the way for a brighter, healthier future, lifting the burden of cancer and improving lives across the globe.

4.5. The Future of Cancer Treatment

The landscape of cancer treatment is rapidly evolving, driven by advances in scientific research, technology, and a deeper understanding of the complexities of cancer biology. As the global incidence of cancer continues to rise, the search for more effective therapies has intensified. This subchapter aims to delve into the exciting prospects for the future of cancer treatment, highlighting innovative strategies, emerging technologies, and the ongoing commitment to patient-centered care.

One of the most promising developments on the horizon is the growing emphasis on personalized medicine. Refining treatments to align with the unique genetic makeup of a patient's tumor allows for more precise therapies that target specific mutations or pathways associated with cancer. The advent of genomic sequencing technologies has enabled researchers and clinicians to analyze tumors at an unprecedented level, uncovering critical insights that inform treatment decisions. In the future, we can anticipate a routine use of genomic profiling in clinical settings, allowing oncologists to tailor therapies based on an individual's tumor biology rather than a one-size-fits-all approach. These advances could lead to improved outcomes and reduced side effects, as patients receive treatments more likely to be effective for their specific cancer type.

In tandem with personalized medicine is the evolution of immunotherapy, which harnesses the body's immune system to combat cancer more effectively. Immune checkpoint inhibitors, CAR T-cell therapy, and personalized cancer vaccines are advancing rapidly through clinical trials and into standard treatment protocols. The future of immunotherapy looks particularly promising, with research focused on overcoming existing limitations, such as tumor resistance and immune tolerance. Combination therapies that pair immunotherapy with traditional treatments like chemotherapy or radiation are being explored to enhance efficacy. Additionally, the potential to develop universal or off-the-shelf immune therapies could democratize access to cutting-edge treatments, offering hope to patients who previously had limited options.

Another exciting area of exploration in future cancer treatment is the use of targeted therapies. The journey from discovery to clinical application has seen the emergence of drugs targeting specific molecular changes that drive cancer progression. As researchers continue identifying critical signaling pathways involved in tumor growth and survival, more targeted agents are becoming available. This approach minimizes damage to normal cells while maximizing the therapeutic impact on cancer cells, heralding a new era of precision oncology. The increasingly comprehensive understanding of cancer genomics ensures that targeted treatments will become an integral part of the cancer treatment landscape.

Furthermore, the integration of artificial intelligence (AI) and machine learning into cancer research promises to reshape diagnostics and treatment planning. AI algorithms that analyze vast datasets from clinical studies, patient records, and genomic information are being trained to identify patterns that may elude traditional analytical methods. These technologies have the potential to facilitate earlier detection of cancer, predict treatment responses, and even assist in designing individualized treatment regimens based on predictive modeling.

Additionally, the field of liquid biopsies offers a glimpse into the future of non-invasive diagnostics. By analyzing circulating tumor DNA (ctDNA) and other biomarkers found in blood samples, liquid biopsies can provide real-time insights into tumor dynamics, treatment efficacy, and disease progression. This innovation could significantly improve the monitoring of patients undergoing treatment, enabling healthcare providers to adjust therapy based on measurable changes rather than relying solely on traditional imaging methods. As research continues to validate these approaches, liquid biopsies may become standard in assessing treatment response and detecting relapses early.

The future of cancer treatment is not limited to new drugs or techniques; it also involves a comprehensive approach to holistic patient care. The importance of integrating psychological support, nutritional guidance, and social services into cancer treatment plans cannot be overstated. As the healthcare community increasingly acknowledges the multidimensional nature of cancer care, models that prioritize comprehensive supportive services will likely become foundational in cancer treatment protocols. Creating partnerships between oncologists, mental health professionals, nutritionists, and palliative care specialists will help address the diverse needs of patients, fostering healing beyond the confines of traditional medicine.

Moreover, enhancing patient and caregiver education will empower individuals to become active participants in their care. Encouraging open dialogues about treatment options, potential side effects, and lifestyle modifications can help patients make informed decisions about their health. In light of prolific misinformation about alternative remedies, such as apricot seeds, establishing channels for credible health communication will be crucial in guiding patients through the complexities of treatment choice.

As we look ahead, it is vital to address the barriers to healthcare access that exist in many regions. Innovations in telemedicine, mobile health technologies, and community outreach initiatives will play an essential role in enhancing access to cancer care, particularly for underserved populations. Bridging the gap in healthcare equity ensures that advancements in cancer treatment benefit all individuals, irrespective of geographic, economic, or social factors.

In conclusion, the future of cancer treatment is poised for transformative change driven by scientific innovation, a commitment to patient-centeredness, and collaboration among interdisciplinary teams. As we embrace the interplay of personalized medicine, immunotherapy, targeted treatments, AI, and holistic care, we move closer to a world where cancer is not a death sentence but a manageable chronic condition. The continued advancement in research, combined with efforts to ensure equitable access to emerging therapies, will be paramount in shaping a future where patients have the tools, support, and options to navigate their cancer journey successfully. Ultimately, the overarching goal remains steadfast: to conquer cancer through the fusion of knowledge, compassion, and transformative research.

5. Apricots: Delightful Fruit or Health Hazard?

5.1. The Nutritional Value of Apricots

The nutritional value of apricots is a vital topic that sheds light on this delightful fruit's intrinsic health benefits while distinguishing it from the contentious narrative surrounding its seeds. Apricots (Prunus armeniaca) are small, orange-hued fruits that not only add a burst of flavor to various culinary dishes but are also rich in essential vitamins and minerals. Their profile is compelling enough to warrant attention, particularly as discussions around cancer treatment and prevention evolve.

One of the standout features of apricots is their impressive vitamin content. They are particularly high in vitamin A, primarily in the form of provitamin A carotenoids like beta-carotene. This nutrient plays a significant role in maintaining healthy eyesight, supporting the immune system, and promoting skin health. A single serving of apricots can provide a considerable portion of the daily recommended intake of vitamin A, highlighting their importance not just as a snack but as a functional food contributing to overall well-being.

Moreover, apricots are excellent sources of vitamins C and E, both potent antioxidants that help protect the body against oxidative stress. Vitamin C is particularly known for its role in collagen synthesis, immunity enhancement, and iron absorption. In addition, the antioxidant properties of vitamin E can assist in reducing inflammation and bolstering skin health. Regular consumption of apricots can thus contribute to a robust nutritional profile that supports various bodily functions and overall health.

Fiber is another remarkable aspect of apricots' nutritional value. These fruits are rich in dietary fiber, which is vital for promoting healthy digestion. Adequate fiber intake supports regular bowel movements by adding bulk to the stool and helps prevent constipation. It is also associated with lower cholesterol levels, improved blood sugar control, and a reduced risk of gastrointestinal disorders. Consequently, apricots can play a role in maintaining digestive health, contributing to the overall approach to diet and wellness.

The mineral content of apricots further enhances their nutritional appeal. They are a good source of potassium, which is essential for maintaining heart health, regulating blood pressure, and supporting muscle function. Potassium is a vital electrolyte that helps balance fluids in the body, and its presence in apricots makes them an excellent snack for those looking to optimize hydration and electrolyte levels, particularly during hot weather or after exercise.

Additionally, apricots contain trace amounts of other critical minerals, such as magnesium, iron, and calcium. Magnesium is crucial for numerous biochemical reactions in the body, including energy production and muscle contraction, while iron is vital for the formation of red blood cells and the transport of oxygen throughout the body. The presence of these minerals adds another dimension to the health benefits associated with apricots, making them a valuable inclusion in a balanced diet.

The health benefits of apricots extend beyond just their raw form; they can be enjoyed fresh, dried, or in various preparations such as jams, jellies, and sauces. Dried apricots, in particular, maintain many of their nutritional benefits and can provide a concentrated source of vitamins and minerals, making them a powerful addition to snacks or meal preparations.

Despite the abundant health benefits associated with apricots, it is crucial to differentiate between the nutritional advantages of the fruit itself and the potentially harmful aspects of apricot seeds. The seeds contain amygdalin, a compound that can convert to cyanide in the body, posing significant health risks when consumed in unregulated amounts. This dichotomy emphasizes the need for careful consideration when discussing apricot seeds and their purported health claims.

In summary, apricots stand out as a nutrient-dense fruit that provides an array of vitamins, minerals, and health-promoting compounds. Their rich nutritional value makes them an excellent choice for enhancing diet quality and supporting overall health. However, as discussions about apricot seeds continue to swirl, it is vital to approach any claims regarding their health benefits with skepticism and rely on rigorous scientific evidence. The focus should remain on the fruit itself, which offers impressive health benefits without the risks associated with its seeds, providing a sweet and nutritious addition to a balanced diet.

5.2. Cyanide Poison: The Kernel Inside the Seed

Cyanide poison, in the context of apricot seeds, unveils a narrative woven with hope, danger, and misconception. At the heart of this conversation lies amygdalin, a compound found in the seeds of apricots and other related fruits, which has garnered attention due to its association with cancer treatment. The allure of a natural solution to a devastating disease can overshadow the potential risks associated with its consumption and lead to a cascade of misinformation.

Amygdalin, often misidentified as vitamin B17, is perceived by some to be a miracle cure for cancer. Proponents of this belief argue that the body metabolizes amygdalin into cyanide which supposedly targets cancer cells, sparing healthy ones. This narrative has penetrated public consciousness, encouraging people to consume apricot seeds and other sources of amygdalin in hopes of battling cancer. However, this simplistic explanation fails to recognize the biochemical reality underlying cyanide metabolism and its acute toxicity.

Cyanide is a potent poison that inhibits the body's ability to use oxygen, effectively leading to cellular suffocation. The consumption of apricot seeds in substantial quantities poses a significant risk, as the amygdalin content can yield dangerous levels of cyanide in the body. While the human body does possess enzymatic pathways capable of detoxifying smaller doses of cyanide, large amounts can overwhelm these systems, leading to poisoning symptoms that can be life-threatening.

Research and clinical observations provide a stark contrast to the optimistic claims surrounding apricot seeds. Documented cases of cyanide poisoning from apricot kernels have emerged, often presenting with a range of symptoms: headache, nausea, vomiting, difficulty breathing, and, in severe circumstances, seizures and loss of consciousness. Some victims have suffered fatal consequences due to the consumption of these seeds, which underscores the critical need for public awareness regarding the dangers they pose when consumed in unregulated, high doses.

The scientific community's consensus has been decisive: while apricot seeds may have a place in the realm of nutrition, the claim that they serve as a viable cancer treatment is not only unsubstantiated but also hazardous. Regulatory bodies, including the U.S. Food and Drug Administration (FDA), have acknowledged these risks and have issued warnings against the consumption of apricot seeds for therapeutic purposes. Additionally, many countries have banned the sale of amygdalin as a treatment for cancer unless it is strictly controlled.

To effectively combat misinformation surrounding apricot seeds and their toxic potential, it is imperative to promote research-driven educational initiatives aimed at empowering individuals to evaluate health claims critically. The juxtaposition of desirable narratives—natural cures invoking hope—against scientifically validated risks must be skillfully navigated, fostering a culture that values evidence-based health practices over alluring simplifications.

As we strive to understand the complex interplay of health information available today, it is essential to provide comprehensive insights into the risks and realities associated with substances claiming to offer miraculous benefits. Engaging communities in discussing the implications of consuming apricot seeds while advocating for informed health choices can reshape the discourse surrounding alternative treatments. This nuanced approach will not only safeguard public health but also encourage a more discerning attitude towards purported natural remedies, empowering individuals to navigate their health choices with knowledge and caution.

In closing, while the apricot may be cherished for its delightful flavor and nutritional profile, it is crucial to exercise caution regarding its seeds. The narrative of apricot seeds as a simple solution to complex health issues must be meticulously examined, stripped of romantic notions and grounded in rigorous scientific understanding. By elevating awareness of the substantial risks involved with cyanide poisoning, we can begin to unravel the web of misinformation that surrounds these unregulated products and move towards a future informed by knowledge, safety, and health advocacy.

5.3. The Origins of the Apricot Seed Myth

The origins of the apricot seed myth trace back through a confluence of historical, cultural, and scientific narratives, collectively weaving a tale that both captivates and misleads. Embedded within this myth is the alluring idea that a simple, natural remedy could provide power-ful healing benefits—specifically targeting one of humanity's gravest challenges: cancer. This notion has taken root over decades, shaped by anecdotes, the appeal of naturalism, and a distrust of conventional medicine.

The early origins of the claim surrounding apricot seeds can be linked to the broader historical context of natural remedies used throughout human civilization. Ancient cultures relied on plants and herbal medicines for health and healing, fostering notions that certain fruits and their seeds held miraculous properties. The apricot tree itself has origins in ancient China, spreading to the Mediterranean regions and beyond, where its fruits were prized not only for their taste but also for their supposed health benefits. Folklore around natural cures often elevates the narrative of seeds and nuts—believing that components of fruit sometimes have protective or curative properties.

As time progressed into the mid-20th century, the narrative evolved further with the advent of a more scientifically attuned fascination with the compounds found in nature, particularly as modern medicine began to question its efficacy. A significant turning point occurred with the introduction of "vitamin B17," a term often used interchange-ably with amygdalin, a compound found in apricot seeds, while the term itself is largely a marketing invention with no official nutritional designation. The promotion of amygdalin as a health supplement began in the 1950s, primarily through the works of certain alternative medicine proponents who posited that it could serve as a viable treatment for cancer.

One critical figure in this myth's rise was Ernst T. Krebs Jr., a biochemist who suggested that amygdalin could prevent or cure cancer. This premise was rooted in a mixture of dismissal of conventional cancer treatments and an overromanticized trust in natural products. Krebs's assertions lacked rigorous scientific validation but were compelling enough to garner a following among those looking for alternatives to the increasingly industrialized pharmaceutical landscape.

The intertwining of the apricot seed myth with alternative medicine took a firm hold in the 1970s, when marketing campaigns began to flourish. The term "Laetrile," derived from amygdalin, emerged during this period, further solidifying a narrative that positioned this compound as a miracle cure for cancer. Laetrile became associated with various advocacy groups and individuals, appealing to those disillusioned with traditional cancer treatments, where patients often faced invasive procedures and harsh side effects.

The popularity of Laetrile and the perceived benefits of apricot seeds were energized by anecdotal testimonials from patients claiming remarkable recoveries after incorporating these seeds into their diets. These success stories echoed through natural health channels, emphasizing hope and the tantalizing notion of reclaiming one's health without conventional interventions. However, the organic nature of these claims often obscured underlying health risks—particularly the significant danger posed by cyanogenic compounds present in apricot seeds, which can lead to cyanide poisoning when consumed in large amounts.

The enduring appeal of the apricot seed myth lies within deeper sociocultural dynamics, including a widespread skepticism towards pharmaceutical companies—perceived as profit-driven entities that may overlook patient welfare. This skepticism has woven itself into the fabric of alternative medicine, where individuals can seek empowerment and agency in their health choices through natural alternatives, despite lacking empirical validation.

This myth has persisted into the digital age, proliferating through social media platforms and wellness blogs, where anecdotal evidence and testimonies can easily escalate and root themselves in popular narratives. The combination of emotionally charged narratives, cultural heritage surrounding natural remedies, and distrust in conventional medicine has created fertile ground for the apricot seed myth to thrive, often overshadowing scientific inquiry and cautionary tales from the medical community.

As we endeavor to unpack the origins of this myth, it is crucial to recognize the complex interplay of historical traditions, cultural beliefs, and emerging narratives that continue to shape public perception and health decisions. The apricot seed myth exemplifies how misinformation can flourish amidst genuine desires for health and healing, calling for critical scrutiny and education to navigate the waters of health information effectively. In doing so, we can honor the legacy of ancient wellness practices while prioritizing the safety and efficacy informed by rigorous scientific evidence.

5.4. Documented Cases of Apricot Seed Poisoning

In exploring the documented cases of apricot seed poisoning, we can uncover a concerning narrative that underscores the significant risks associated with unregulated consumption of these seeds. Apricot seeds, which contain amygdalin—a naturally occurring compound often touted by some as a cancer cure—have been connected to instances of cyanide poisoning. The stories and evidence surrounding such cases serve as critical reminders of the dangers posed by unverified health recommendations and the need for cautious scrutiny in the face of appealing natural remedies.

Historically, the allure of apricot seeds has drawn various individuals to incorporate them into their diets in hopes of reaping supposed health benefits. Promoters of apricot seeds have often claimed that their consumption can combat cancer, attributing these claims to the presence of amygdalin, which is sometimes misleadingly referred to as vitamin B17. However, emerging reports of adverse health effects have painted a starkly different picture, challenging the romanticized narratives surrounding these seeds.

One well-documented case involves an individual who consumed large quantities of apricot seeds as part of a personal health regimen aimed at treating a diagnosed illness. Shortly after ingestion, the individual began experiencing symptoms consistent with cyanide poisoning, which may include severe headaches, nausea, vomiting, difficulty breathing, and decreased consciousness. Medical intervention was required, and the individual was ultimately treated in a healthcare facility, where they underwent detoxification procedures to combat the toxic effects of cyanide.

Several similar cases have emerged over the years, particularly among individuals drawn to alternative health methodologies and unregulated natural products, where the risks may not be adequately communicated. In one notable instance, a group of individuals affiliated with an alternative health website shared testimonials praising apricot seeds for their purported health benefits. Subsequently, multiple members of that group reported severe symptoms as a direct result of consuming apricot seeds in excessive quantities. As medical professionals evaluated these cases, it became increasingly clear that serious health risks were associated with the consumption of these seeds, prompting consultations on the importance of health education that emphasizes evidence-based information.

In addition to individual accounts, public health agencies and poison control centers have documented a range of adverse reactions linked to apricot seed consumption. Some reports detail instances of patients requiring emergency medical intervention due to catastrophic levels of cyanide in their systems. Symptoms of acute cyanide poisoning include but are not limited to cardiac arrest, respiratory failure, and seizures. While mild cases may lead to more manageable symptoms, the variability of individual tolerance—and particularly the potential for cumulative toxicity from overconsumption—makes the risks inherent and serious.

The potential for cyanide poisoning is particularly alarming considering the lack of standardized guidance around the consumption of apricot seeds. The absence of regulation regarding the sale of these seeds as health products can lead consumers to underestimate the risks associated with their consumption. This is compounded by the fact that individuals may unknowingly consume large numbers of seeds, attracted by anecdotal claims of their health-promoting effects.

Furthermore, regulatory agencies like the FDA have taken action to communicate the dangers of apricot seeds. Despite some anecdotal praises for the seeds as natural remedies, the consensus is clear: the risks of cyanide poisoning far outweigh any unsubstantiated benefits touted by proponents. In several countries, the marketing and distribution of products containing apricot seeds have been restricted due to the lack of evidence supporting their safety and efficacy, particularly in medicinal contexts.

In summary, the documented cases of apricot seed poisoning illuminate a critical cautionary tale regarding unverified health claims. As individuals seek natural remedies and alternatives to conventional medicine, it is paramount to remain informed about the potential consequences—especially for products that lack rigorous scientific validation. The stories of those who have suffered poisoning serve as stark reminders of the importance of public health education, advocating for informed choices guided by credible research rather than unfounded claims. Moving forward, promoting awareness around the risks associated with apricot seeds can help ensure healthier choices and better protections for consumers, allowing individuals to empower their health journeys without exposing themselves to avoidable dangers.

5.5. Scientific Community's Consensus

The scientific community's consensus regarding the use of apricot seeds as a cancer treatment is rooted firmly in rigorous research and extensive clinical evidence. When popular claims surrounding natural remedies gain traction, it becomes essential for health professionals and researchers to investigate the validity of these claims through the lens of empirical data. In the case of apricot seeds, the recommendations they promote often tout the supposed anti-cancer properties linked to the amygdalin they contain.

Amygdalin, once popularly misrepresented as vitamin B17, has been marketed as a miracle cure for various cancers. However, the scientific community has thoroughly examined these claims, and the results paint a decidedly different picture. Extensive studies exploring the efficacy of amygdalin have, time and again, demonstrated that there is insufficient evidence supporting the idea that consuming apricot seeds or amygdalin can effectively treat cancer. Open clinical trials and peer-reviewed articles fail to show that amygdalin offers any significant therapeutic benefit in combating malignancies. Instead, these studies have often revealed the potential for adverse health reactions, notably cyanide poisoning.

The consensus has been bolstered by corroborating statements from reputable organizations such as the American Cancer Society, the U.S. Food and Drug Administration (FDA), and various global health authorities. These institutions emphasize the importance of relying on scientifically validated cancer treatments rather than unproven natural remedies. They point to the inherent dangers posed by high levels of cyanide present in apricot seeds as a reason for caution. Reports of severe poisoning stemming from excessive consumption highlight the risks involved and demonstrate why the medical community remains skeptical regarding claims that promote apricot seeds as a viable treatment option.

Furthermore, the scientific consensus extends to concerns about the dissemination of misinformation. The spread of unproven health claims can hinder patients from accessing effective treatments, as individuals may forego established medical protocols in favor of these alluring yet dangerous alternatives. Engaging with the narratives surrounding apricot seeds showcases the difficulty health experts face when challenging deeply ingrained beliefs about natural remedies. In addressing the topic, it becomes vital to clarify the risks associated with apricot seeds while reiterating the necessity of evidence-based medicine.

In dealing with misinformation, researchers and clinicians advocate for increased public health education campaigns designed to clarify the true nature of these claims. Through the dissemination of accurate, research-backed information, the scientific community aims to illuminate the discrepancies between anecdotal evidence and empirical data. Educating the public about the importance of informed decision-making and the potential harm of relying on unregulated remedies like apricot seeds stands as a crucial objective in public health advocacy.

As we move forward in discussing the use of apricot seeds and their purported health benefits, it is clear that the scientific community maintains a firm stance grounded in research and factual evidence. Individuals grappling with cancer or other significant health concerns should be encouraged to seek guidance from qualified medical professionals and avoid unverified treatments that could jeopardize their health. The road to wellness must prioritize safety, evidence, and the effective integration of scientifically validated treatment modalities, ensuring that lives can be saved and health can be preserved.

6. Unpacking the Health Claims: Separating Fact From Fiction

6.1. The Lure of Simple Solutions

The quest for simple solutions to complex problems has pervaded human history, especially in the realm of health and wellness. The allure of discovering a "magic bullet"—a single remedy carrying the promise of effectively tackling intricate health challenges—speaks to our innate desire for quick fixes. This notion remains profoundly alluring, particularly when confronted with life-threatening diseases like cancer. The idea that a common, everyday item like apricot seeds could potentially harbor the power to combat cancer exemplifies the powerful pull of these simple solutions. However, beneath the gleaming façade of such narratives lies a more complex reality, replete with medical misinformation, unregulated claims, and ethical dilemmas.

At the heart of this narrative is the psychological comfort found in natural remedies. Many individuals grapple with feelings of helplessness when faced with dire health conditions, compelling them to search for alternative solutions outside traditional medicine. In this context, apricot seeds and their purported benefits become emblematic of a broader desire for agency in health choices. The assertion that a natural substance could offer a reprieve from a dire diagnosis appeals not only as a beacon of hope but also as a path to reclaiming control over one's health. This emotive connection to natural cures often outweighs the rational considerations surrounding their efficacy and safety.

The romanticized image of natural remedies plays into a narrative that is easily digestible and compelling. In a world dominated by skepticism towards pharmaceutical companies and the perceived impersonal nature of medical treatments, the idea of a simple, organic solution resonates strongly. The notion that "nature knows best" feeds into this psychological draw, allowing individuals to cling to the belief that the right remedy is simply a seed or a root away, often obscuring the nuances of rigorous scientific scrutiny. This reinforces a collective yearning for simplicity in a complex arena, where formulating nuanced understanding can feel intellectually and emotionally taxing.

Moreover, these appealing narratives are further reinforced through the lens of social influence. Testimonials from survivors or self-proclaimed health advocates asserting miraculous recoveries after incorporating apricot seeds into their medicinal regimen encapsulate this dynamic well. Such anecdotes, peppered with emotional weight, communicate a strong social bond; individuals who share these narratives act as informal health advocates, crafting a compelling case for the efficacy of the natural remedy. The persuasive power of these personal stories can quickly overshadow the vital need for evidence-based medicine, leaving many vulnerable to misinformation.

In the digital age, the propagation of such simplistic narratives is especially amplified. Various online platforms serve as echo chambers where enthusiastic endorsements of natural remedies, like apricot seeds, can proliferate without critical engagement. This milieu allows for the rapid dissemination of unverified information, contributing to the diversification of health beliefs that often contradict sound scientific evidence. The risk here is profound: as beliefs founded on hope and naturalism take root, individuals may bypass conventional treatments, leading to potentially catastrophic health outcomes.

While the lure of simple solutions undeniably captures attention, it is crucial to temper this allure with sober realities. Fostering health literacy becomes paramount as we navigate this dense landscape. Empowering individuals to distinguish between anecdotal claims and scientifically validated findings equips them to make informed choices about their health. Education plays a critical role in unraveling the intricate threads of misinformation, enabling individuals to maintain a discerning eye towards health claims that promise seemingly magical outcomes.

Furthermore, the responsibility lies heavily with health advocates, practitioners, and regulators to create a balanced narrative around health choices. Promoting transparency about the limitations and risks associated with alternatives such as apricot seeds—chiefly the danger of cyanide toxicity linked with their consumption—must take precedence over romanticism. By providing accessible educational resources, we can pave the way for communities to engage in informed discussions about health remedies, empowering them to navigate choices wisely.

Ultimately, the journey from yearning for simple solutions to cultivating wise health choices is a complex, multifaceted endeavor. While the desire for natural, uncomplicated remedies is deeply ingrained in human health narratives, the challenge remains to root these discussions in truth, caution, and scientific inquiry. By embracing both the allure of nature's bounty and the rigor of science, we can navigate these paths towards wellness with clarity, responsibility, and integrity, ensuring that hope never overruns health. In this delicate equilibrium lies the promise of sustainable health practices that cherish both ancient wisdom and empirical validation, guiding society towards a future where informed choices reign supreme.

6.2. Busting the Myths Around B17 and Laetrile

The narrative surrounding apricot seeds and their association with cancer treatment is imbued with a multitude of myths and misconceptions, notably including the popular but misguided belief in vitamin B17 and its purported healing properties. At the center of this discourse lies laetrile, a compound derived from amygdalin commonly extracted from apricot seeds, which has garnered attention as an alleged natural anti-cancer agent. However, the sweeping claims made in favor of laetrile as a miracle cure demand critical examination, as they often rest on shaky foundations devoid of scientific validation.

The origins of the myth surrounding laetrile can be traced back to the late 1950s and 1960s, when proponents began asserting its efficacy in treating cancer—a notion primarily fueled by anecdotal reports rather than robust clinical evidence. The claims of laetrile being an alternative treatment began to gain traction among individuals disillusioned by conventional cancer therapies, which were often characterized by severe side effects and invasive procedures. This disenchantment with mainstream treatments set the stage for natural remedies, including laetrile, to thrive as appealing alternatives.

At the heart of the advocacy for laetrile is the assertion that amygdalin, once ingested, metabolizes into cyanide, which proponents claimed could specifically target and destroy cancer cells while leaving healthy cells unharmed. This claim, however, was primarily predicated on oversimplified biochemical assumptions and fundamentally flawed reasoning. The reality is that cyanide is a potent poison that will adversely affect all cellular structures, creating the very real risk of cyanide poisoning.

Numerous studies have evaluated the effects of amygdalin and laetrile, concluding that there is no substantial evidence to support the efficacy of these compounds in effectively treating cancer or improving patient outcomes. The scientific literature overwhelmingly reflects a consensus that the risks associated with these products far outweigh any supposed benefits. Rather than being an effective treatment, laetrile has led to serious health complications—including fatalities from cyanide poisoning—highlighting the urgent need for stringent regulatory oversight and public health education.

The lack of regulatory endorsement for laetrile serves as an important reminder of the ethical responsibilities held within the realm of alternative treatments. In the United States, for example, the Food and Drug Administration (FDA) has cited laetrile as ineffective and dangerous, providing further evidence that consumer protection measures are warranted in relation to unverified and potentially hazardous products.

As society delves deeper into the narratives surrounding alternative therapies, it is vital to confront the myths perpetuated around substances like laetrile and amygdalin directly. Combating the allure of oversimplified solutions with factual evidence is crucial in shaping public perception and ensuring individuals make informed health choices. The stories of patients who have pinned their hopes on apricot seeds and laetrile should not only be met with empathy, but also with rigorous scrutiny of the scientific data, which must underscore the risks involved.

Education and awareness are paramount as we navigate the complex interplay of alternative medicine beliefs and scientific realities. Public health initiatives should focus on disseminating accurate information about cancer treatments that delves into factual evaluations rather than sensationalized claims. This also involves fostering dialogues between the scientific community and the public, effectively bridging knowledge gaps to encourage critical thinking in health decisions.

The myth of laetrile serves as a powerful reminder of the implications of alternative treatments promoted without sufficient evidence— underscoring the necessity for comprehensive evaluation and robust regulatory measures. For individuals grappling with the complexities of cancer treatment, a clear understanding of the realities surround- ing apricot seeds, laetrile, and the broader landscape of alternative medicine will empower them to make informed choices that prioritize safety and efficacy over the allure of unsubstantiated promises. In doing so, we can navigate the intricate world of health information with caution and discernment, ultimately fostering a culture that values verified science and patient safety above all else.

6.3. Media Narratives vs. Scientific Evidence

Media narratives play a significant role in shaping public perception of health-related issues, especially concerning controversial topics such as the use of apricot seeds as an alternative cancer treatment. The appeal of these narratives often rests on emotional resonance rather than factual accuracy, leading individuals to prioritize anec- dotal evidence over rigorous scientific inquiry. This phenomenon is particularly evident in the case of apricot seeds, where the belief in their cancer-fighting properties, based on individual testimonials and social media stories, overshadows clear scientific evidence to the contrary.

Media outlets, influenced by the compelling nature of personal stories, can amplify claims about natural remedies without adequately presenting the associated risks or the scientific consensus. For example, sensationalized reports might highlight miraculous recoveries attributed to apricot seed consumption, thereby fostering a narrative that prioritizes hope over reason. Such media portrayals contribute to a fertile ground for misinformation to flourish, often resulting in the propagation of false beliefs about the efficacy of unproven treatments within the broader public.

The effectiveness of any health communication is also intricately tied to the methodologies employed by various media platforms. Traditional media, such as television and newspapers, have a distinct capacity to reach wide audiences, yet they sometimes portray health information simplistically, often resorting to misleading headlines that can evoke fear or false hope. The entertainment factor prevalent in modern news cycles can lead to a focus on drama at the expense of clarity, undermining the very ethos of responsible health reporting. Meanwhile, the rise of digital media allows for rapid dissemination and virality of unverified claims, demonstrating both the benefits and challenges present in the digital landscape.

Social media platforms represent a double-edged sword in the discourse surrounding health. They offer spaces for peer support and community sharing, where individuals can discover alternative solutions and advice. However, these platforms also propagate misinformation rapidly, as viral trends can emerge without critical examination. Health-related hashtags are often co-opted by businesses looking to capitalize on consumer interest, reinforcing the narratives that prioritize profit over safety. The algorithms used by social media networks favor content that garners high engagement, often leading to sensational stories being promoted while more factual, yet mundane, content is buried.

Moreover, the allure of simple solutions can exacerbate the issue, as people tend to gravitate towards narratives that offer quick fixes to complex problems. The notion that something as common as an apricot seed could hold the key to combating cancer is captivating, naturally leading individuals to dismiss more nuanced discussions about cancer treatment grounded in scientific research and evidence. The perception of crisis in the face of a severe illness generates a willingness to embrace potential cures, often at the risk of compromising informed decision-making.

In this age of rapid information turnover, the scientific community faces immense challenges in countering skewed media narratives. Robust communication strategies must be implemented to ensure that accurate information reaches the public efficiently and effectively. This includes proactive outreach efforts from healthcare professionals, leveraging their credibility to provide balanced perspectives in public discussions about alternative treatments.

Critical thinking plays an essential role as consumers are tasked with discerning fact from fiction in the deluge of health information. In an environment teeming with mixed messages, readers must cultivate the ability to evaluate claims critically. This is particularly crucial in matters such as the apricot seed narrative, where adherence to anecdotal evidence without scientific backing can pose significant health risks.

Ultimately, the contrast between media narratives and scientific evidence underscores the necessity for a more informed public. As individuals seek health solutions, coherent communication that prioritizes clarity and accuracy is imperative. We must foster an understanding that while stories can inspire, they should not serve as substitutes for empirical research. By advocating for responsible media coverage and empowering individuals with the knowledge to navigate the complexities of health information, we can strive to dismantle the misleading narratives that persist in the public consciousness. The story of apricot seeds exemplifies the broader discourse on health and wellness, serving as a reminder of the critical intersection where media influence and scientific inquiry must converge for the benefit of public health.

6.4. The Role of Confirmation Bias

In the vast arena of health and wellness, confirmation bias plays a significant role in shaping individuals' beliefs and decision-making processes regarding alternative treatments, especially concerning natural remedies like apricot seeds for cancer. This cognitive bias refers to the tendency of people to favor information that confirms their preexisting beliefs while dismissing or undervaluing evidence that contradicts these beliefs. Within the context of healthcare and disease management, confirmation bias can have profound implications, often leading individuals away from evidence-based medicine and towards unverified alternatives that promise miraculous cures.

The allure of apricot seeds as a potential cancer treatment exemplifies how confirmation bias can manifest. Those who gravitate towards the idea of apricot seeds as a viable remedy are often already predisposed to believe in the efficacy of natural treatments, which can stem from personal experiences, cultural beliefs, or emotional needs. When individuals come across anecdotal testimonials about someone experiencing relief or improvement in their cancer symptoms after consuming apricot seeds, they are more likely to accept this information as validation of their beliefs. The compelling narrative of someone overcoming illness using a simple, natural solution resonates deeply with their desires, causing them to embrace these claims enthusiastically.

Conversely, individuals who prioritize scientific evidence and traditional medical practices may encounter scientific studies that highlight the dangers associated with apricot seed consumption, including the risks of cyanide poisoning. However, confirmation bias can lead them to either disregard these findings or reinterpret them to fit within their existing framework of understanding. For example, they may rationalize the risks as contingent upon dosage or argue that negative outcomes are exceptions rather than the rule. This selective reading and internal reasoning create an echo chamber reinforcing their preferred narratives, making it increasingly challenging to engage in constructive dialogue that urges critical examination of their beliefs.

The role of social media further amplifies the effects of confirmation bias, as individuals typically engage with like-minded communities that share and propagate similar health narratives. The prevalence of influencers promoting health claims about apricot seeds can create viral trends that solidify bias-based thinking within these spaces. Support groups, blogs, and forums amplifying personal stories of success or recovery can overshadow the counterarguments presented by healthcare professionals and researchers. As members of these communities interact, sharing their experiences reinforces beliefs in apricot seeds' efficacy, creating a culture where dissenting opinions struggle to gain traction.

Additionally, the influence of cognitive dissonance is closely tied to confirmation bias. When individuals are confronted with evidence that contradicts their beliefs about apricot seeds, they experience discomfort or dissonance. To alleviate this psychological tension, they may choose to dismiss or rationalize the conflicting evidence, reinforcing their preconceived notions. This cycle perpetuates misinformation and creates an environment resistant to new ideas or reassessments of established beliefs, even when faced with overwhelming scientific consensus that undermines the anecdotal claims.

In navigating the healthcare landscape, it becomes increasingly critical to develop awareness of confirmation bias's impact. Health education campaigns need to address these psychological tendencies, promoting a culture of critical thinking and open discourse about health choices. Encouraging individuals to question their beliefs and seek out diverse perspectives can help cultivate a more nuanced understanding of health information, especially in cases of contentious remedies such as apricot seeds.

Moreover, transparency from healthcare professionals in discussing the limitations and potential risks of alternative treatments is necessary to combat misinformation. Presenting factual information that highlights both supportive and contradictory evidence enables individuals to engage with health claims critically, fostering informed decision-making rooted in science rather than anecdote.

Ultimately, recognizing and understanding the role of confirmation bias is fundamental to evaluating health information effectively. By fostering an environment that prioritizes evidence-based discussions and critical engagement, we can move toward a more informed society that appreciates the complexities of health choices without succumbing to the allure of simplistic narratives. The challenge lies in bridging the gap between deeply held beliefs and scientific inquiry, encouraging a balanced perspective that can lead to more prudent health choices and ultimately, improved outcomes for all.

6.5. Reflections on Public Perception

In attempting to understand public perception, it is critical to explore how societal beliefs and attitudes evolve in response to health messages, particularly regarding alternative treatments like apricot seeds for cancer. The allure of natural remedies reflects a complex interplay of historical trust in nature, cultural beliefs about health, and the emotional narratives that accompany personal experiences. At its root, public perception is shaped by both the information available and the psychological factors influencing how individuals engage with that information.

Historically, there has been a profound shift towards natural remedies, often reflecting a reaction to the perceived shortcomings of conventional medicine. For many, the journey through the medical system—characterized by procedures or pharmaceuticals—can be disillusioning, fostering a yearning for simpler, more holistic solutions. Alternative therapies often embody a romantic ideal: the notion that nature holds the key to healing, and that solutions can be found in unprocessed, familiar sources like fruits, herbs, and seeds. This aligns neatly with widely held beliefs that "natural" equates to "safe" and "good," thereby bolstering public interest in often unproven remedies.

The consumption of apricot seeds serves as a poignant case study in this phenomenon. While the seeds have been touted in some circles as a potential cancer treatment due to the presence of amygdalin, claims made about their efficacy have been met with skepticism from medical professionals. Nevertheless, the personal testimonials of individuals who believe they have benefited from these seeds form a compelling narrative that can overshadow scientific discourse. Such testimonials capitalize on emotional appeal—they tell stories of hope, recovery, and empowerment, resonating with those who may feel powerless against serious illness.

Moreover, confirmation bias plays a significant role in shaping how individuals interpret health information about apricot seeds. When presented with evidence supporting the idea that these seeds can fight cancer, those already inclined to believe in the efficacy of natural remedies may disproportionately seek out and emphasize data that aligns with their existing beliefs. This tendency can create echo chambers, particularly through social media platforms, where like-minded individuals amplify their convictions and bolster their faith in alternative therapies, often to the detriment of critical evaluation.

The internet has reshaped the landscape of health information, empowering individuals with unprecedented access to diverse view-points but also creating venues for misinformation. Online communities, blogs, and social media have become fertile grounds for alternative narratives that may lack scientific backing. As public perception becomes increasingly influenced by the proliferation of anecdotal evidence, crucial distinctions between empirical science and personal experience blur, with individuals often choosing to disregard conflicting scientific evidence.

Furthermore, cultural factors play a fundamental role in the sustaining of mythologies around remedies like apricot seeds. In many cultures, there exists a rich tradition of herbalism and the use of plants for medicinal purposes, often steeped in folklore. While such practices can provide valuable insights into holistic approaches to health, they can also lead to the perpetuation of unverified health claims when tradition is prioritized over evidence. The tension between modern medical understanding and traditional practices underscores the need for effective communication strategies that resonate with various cultural beliefs while also promoting informed decision-making grounded in science.

Public perception is also inherently tied to the very nature of health communication. Messages conveyed through various channels —health campaigns, news articles, social media updates—play critical roles in shaping attitudes towards health practices. Emotional narratives often dominate these messages, attaching personal stories to health claims. This emotional appeal can make claims about natural remedies compelling, but the oversimplification inherent in such narratives often fails to account for the complexities of disease and treatment, leaving the public misinformed or misled.

In confronting the public's perception of apricot seeds as a potential cure for cancer, it is vital to ensure that health communication prioritizes clarity, accuracy, and contextual understanding. Efforts should be made to bridge the gap between traditional beliefs and modern science, fostering dialogues that respect cultural practices while advocating for evidence-based health choices. Enhancing public health literacy is paramount, equipping individuals with the tools necessary to navigate the myriad of health claims they encounter, allowing them to distinguish fact from fiction.

Moreover, continued engagement with communities that hold traditional beliefs around health can help build trust and understanding. Collaborative efforts between health professionals and community leaders can provide platforms for discussions around alternative therapies, promoting safe practices while addressing misconceptions.

In conclusion, reflections on public perception reveal a multifaceted relationship between belief, experience, and information. The allure of natural remedies like apricot seeds for cancer reflects a broader societal desire for hope amid uncertainty, intertwined with cultural narratives about healing. However, as we seek to empower individuals to make informed choices about their health, it is critical that narrative simplicity gives way to complexity—acknowledging the intricate balance between tradition, emotion, and scientific evidence. By fostering critical dialogues, promoting health literacy, and bridging cultural divides, we can ensure that personal beliefs do not overshadow the imperative of safety and efficacy in health decision-making.

7. Regulatory Perspectives and Global Responses

7.1. The FDA's Stance on Apricot Seeds

The FDA has taken a firm stance on the use of apricot seeds, particularly regarding their purported cancer-fighting properties. In a landscape where anecdotal claims and alternative therapies often proliferate, the role of regulatory bodies like the Food and Drug Administration becomes critical in safeguarding public health and ensuring that consumers are not misled by unsubstantiated remedies. The FDA's position is informed by comprehensive scientific analysis, clinical evidence, and the imperative to prevent potential harm stemming from the consumption of apricot seeds.

At the heart of the FDA's concerns lies the chemical compound amygdalin, often marketed as "vitamin B17" but scientifically recognized as a cyanogenic glycoside. When ingested, amygdalin can release cyanide in the body, a potent toxin that can interfere with the body's ability to use oxygen and may result in serious health consequences, including death. Consequently, the FDA has issued regulatory warnings regarding the consumption of apricot seeds, particularly in quantities that exceed safe limits.

In 2010, the FDA issued a public health advisory cautioning people against the use of apricot kernels for their purported cancer treatment effects, underscoring the lack of scientific evidence that supports such claims. The advisory pointed out that while proponents may allege benefits based on personal testimonials, robust clinical research has found no evidence to substantiate these claims and significant risks associated with high cyanide levels found in apricot seeds. This announcement carries the weight of empirical scrutiny, illustrating the FDA's commitment to prioritizing consumer safety over unfounded health claims.

Moreover, regulatory responses extend beyond U.S. borders, as international health authorities have echoed the FDA's stance. For example, governments and health organizations in various countries, such as Canada and Australia, have similarly raised alarms about the consumption of apricot seeds. In these nations, there is denouncement of the promotion of apricot seeds as a therapeutic product, reflecting a unified global response to the emerging narrative of apricot seeds as a cancer cure. Such responses are rooted in a collaborative effort of public health officials worldwide to combat misinformation and protect consumers from harmful products.

The FDA has also been active in addressing the broader implications of alternative cancer therapies. The rise of unverified treatments poses a considerable challenge in regulating health products, especially those promoted online. The agency encourages healthcare professionals and consumers alike to exercise caution when evaluating claims about natural remedies. The assertion that apricot seeds can cure cancer may not only represent a misunderstanding of cancer biology but also divert patients from seeking effective, evidence-based treatments, thereby affecting their health outcomes.

Simultaneously, the FDA's recommendations urge individuals to engage critically with health information, heightening the need for consumer awareness campaigns that can effectively communicate the risks of unproven therapies. These campaigns are crucial in providing clear, accessible information about the dangers associated with consuming apricot seeds, emphasizing the importance of relying on scientifically validated treatments for cancer.

Legal actions have also emerged surrounding the marketing of apricot seeds and similar products. Some advocates promoting these seeds have faced scrutiny for disseminating misleading claims. Lawsuits and regulatory actions serve as a reminder that while health freedom allows individuals to explore diverse treatments, it must coexist with accountability—that the responsibility of marketers and advocates lies in ensuring consumers receive accurate information.

The path forward, informed by regulatory perspectives, continues to evolve as public health advocates and scientists work to dispel the myths surrounding apricot seeds while empowering individuals with accurate knowledge. Addressing the misconceptions requires multi-faceted strategies, including public education and outreach initiatives aimed at enhancing health literacy. This integrated approach will better equip consumers to make informed health choices and encourage discourse that emphasizes safety and scientific rigor in health decision-making.

In summary, the FDA's stance on apricot seeds reflects a commitment to public health, underpinned by scientific evidence and a clear warning against the consumption of products linked to potential harm. As consumers navigate the complexities of health information, the roles of regulatory authorities become increasingly crucial in guiding individuals towards effective, evidence-based solutions rather than misleading claims. Coordination with global health authorities strives to ensure a united front against misinformation and enhances consumer protection, paving the way for informed health choices and ultimately contributing to improved health outcomes.

7.2. Global Health Authorities and Unified Responses

The influence of global health authorities in shaping unified responses to health threats cannot be overstated. In an era increasingly characterized by misinformation and rapid dissemination of health narratives, organizations such as the World Health Organization (WHO), the Centers for Disease Control and Prevention (CDC), and national health authorities play critical roles in establishing guidelines grounded in robust scientific evidence. Their efforts are vital in addressing public health crises, including the narrative around alternative treatments such as apricot seeds for cancer.

The complexity of health misinformation necessitates a coordinated response from global health authorities. The proliferation of unverified health claims has been accentuated by the internet and social media. These platforms accelerate the spread of narratives that can contradict established scientific knowledge, leading to public confusion and potentially dangerous health decisions. This situation calls for health authorities to step in, providing fact-based information and guidelines to equip the public with the knowledge required to navigate these treacherous waters.

The WHO, in particular, has become a leading voice in advocating for the importance of evidence-based practice in health. Through their extensive research and references to numerous studies, they have issued warnings regarding alternative remedies lacking scientific validation, including apricot seeds. Their resources emphasize safeguarding public health through rigorous scientific inquiry. By making clear statements about the risks associated with unregulated natural products, they aim to protect the populace from the perils of misinformation about supposed cure-alls derived from natural sources.

One of the WHO's significant contributions is the development of frameworks aimed at improving public health communication. Recognizing that effective messaging is crucial during health crises, they offer guidelines that encourage transparency and a commitment to engaging with communities. The importance of fostering trust between public health institutions and the populations they serve remains vital, especially in perpetuating a unified response against alternative treatments that may lure patients away from traditional medical practices.

However, the mission of health authorities extends beyond merely issuing warnings; it involves collaboration with various stakeholders in the health ecosystem. Policymakers, healthcare providers, and educators must work together to strengthen public health responses. This synergy allows for the dissemination of cohesive information, creating a network of awareness that can counteract the effects of misinformation concerning apricot seeds and other alternative treatments. By formulating comprehensive educational campaigns, health authorities can demystify natural remedies, empowering individuals to make informed choices based on solid evidence rather than anecdotal testimonies.

Moreover, the need for culturally-sensitive approaches cannot be overstated. Global health authorities must recognize the diverse beliefs and practices surrounding health within various communities. When addressing the risks associated with practices like consuming apricot seeds, it is essential to engage with these communities respectfully, fostering dialogue that addresses culturally-held views while providing factual, science-backed counterpoints. Building this trust can facilitate more effective public health campaigns and encourage individuals to consider evidence over myth.

Legal measures and regulatory frameworks also offer another layer of response. Global health authorities often work in conjunction with regulatory bodies to monitor the marketing and sale of potential health hazards. The collaborative approach that involves local and international law enforcement can result in stronger positions against entities promoting false health claims, including those surrounding apricot seeds. This legislation not only emphasizes consumer safety but also underscores the importance of accountability among health advocates and businesses that sell health-related products.

The cravings for simple solutions in times of health crises create fertile ground for alternative remedies like apricot seeds to flourish. As health authorities take on the responsibility of unifying global responses, they must continually refine their strategies to combat misinformation effectively. For example, they can leverage digital platforms to disseminate accurate information rapidly, tapping into the accessibility of social media to pre-empt the virality of false claims.

In summary, global health authorities are poised to play an instrumental role in addressing and countering the misconceptions surrounding natural remedies like apricot seeds. Through a combination of research-backed guidelines, effective community engagement, regulatory oversight, and cross-sector collaboration, these organizations can foster a public health environment that prioritizes safety, efficacy, and informed decision-making amidst the confusion that surrounds alternative treatments. As the landscape of health and wellness continues to evolve, sustained efforts from global health authorities remain crucial in ensuring that patients are empowered to make wise health choices grounded in sound scientific evidence.

7.3. Legal Battles Surrounding Alternative Cancer Cures

Legal battles surrounding alternative cancer cures, particularly focusing on apricot seeds, reveal the complex and often contentious interplay of health advocacy, regulatory oversight, and consumer protection. The popular narrative that apricot seeds, rich in amygdalin—often referred to as "vitamin B17"—can serve as a miracle cure for cancer has driven many individuals to seek legal recourse against claims they perceive as misleading or dangerous. These battles are emblematic of a wider struggle between clinical evidence and the allure of alternative remedies that promise hope, which can often lead to harmful health choices.

Historically, as the narrative that apricot seeds can effectively treat cancer gained traction, so too did the commercial market for these seeds. Individuals and companies began marketing apricot seeds as a natural, life-saving remedy with little regard for the scientific community's extensive research debunking these claims. This disregard has led to a series of lawsuits aimed at holding purveyors of apricot seeds accountable for the potential harm caused by their promotion and sale.

One notable legal case arose when a group of patients who believed they had been misled by advertisements emphasized the supposed cancer-fighting potential of apricot seeds. These individuals suffered adverse health effects as a result of consuming the seeds, many experiencing symptoms of cyanide poisoning after exceeding safe consumption levels. The lawsuit highlighted the ethical obligation of sellers to provide accurate information regarding the risks associated with their products, particularly when those products are marketed as health or treatment aids. Legal frameworks in place aim to protect consumers from deceptive advertising practices, and the plaintiffs were determined to seek justice for the physical and emotional harm they experienced.

Another important dimension of legal battles surrounding alternative cancer cures involves regulatory agencies like the U.S. Food and Drug Administration (FDA). The FDA's stance on apricot seeds emphasizes consumer safety and public health. Amid rising concerns about the promotion of these seeds as cancer treatments, the FDA has issued advisories warning against their use due to the inherent risks of cyanide exposure that come with amygdalin metabolism. The agency's involvement showcases the ongoing struggle to regulate alternative health claims effectively while balancing individual freedom and proactive health choices.

Despite the lack of scientific backing for apricot seeds as a safe or effective cancer treatment, the allure persists. The legal implications highlight the responsibilities of those who market such products and the necessity for stricter regulatory measures to discern between legitimate health claims and unfounded rhetoric. When unverified health products are marketed without adequate oversight, consumers are left vulnerable, and this has spurred advocates to push for more stringent consumer protection laws.

The media's role in the proliferation of myths surrounding apricot seeds has further complicated these legal battles. Sensationalized stories of individuals claiming miraculous recoveries through the consumption of apricot seeds often overshadow the factual evidence presented by the scientific community. These narratives can be powerful, drawing individuals toward alternative remedies and away from established medical practices. Legal action has often sought to confront this misinformation, challenging the narratives that promote unproven remedies and pushing for clearer communication that prioritizes safety and efficacy.

Furthermore, international perspectives on apricot seed use reveal variability in legal frameworks and regulatory responses. In some countries, the unregulated sale of apricot seeds has led to stricter controls, while in others, the seeds remain available without oversight. This disparity raises questions about the global responsibility to protect consumers from false claims related to health and wellness, underscoring the need for collaborative approaches among nations to address these issues.

Consumer protection initiatives and awareness campaigns are vital components in combating misinformation surrounding apricot seeds and alternative cancer remedies. Various health advocacy groups have launched educational campaigns to inform the public about the risks associated with unverified treatments, the dangers of cyanide poisoning from apricot seeds, and the importance of relying on evidence-based medicine. These initiatives aim to empower individuals to make informed decisions about their health, ensuring they are equipped with accurate information necessary to navigate the healthcare landscape.

In summary, legal battles surrounding apricot seeds illustrate the complexities of navigating alternative cancer treatment claims. They underscore the critical need for regulatory frameworks that protect consumers from the dangers of unsubstantiated therapies while honoring patients' rights to explore diverse treatment options. As society grapples with the tensions between personal freedom and public health responsibility, continued vigilance in educating consumers about the risks associated with such remedies is essential. By promoting informed decision-making and holding sellers accountable, it becomes possible to strike a balance that prioritizes safety and well-being in the landscape of health choices.

7.4. Consumer Protection and Awareness Campaigns

Consumer protection and awareness campaigns play a critical role in addressing the pervasive issues of misinformation surrounding health choices, particularly concerning alternative cancer treatments like apricot seeds. In an era where information is delivered at lightning speed through multiple channels—social media, blogs, and websites

—consumers are often inundated with conflicting messages. This white noise can create confusion, leading individuals to make health choices based on anecdotal evidence rather than sound scientific principles. Therefore, the responsibility falls upon public health officials, advocacy groups, and healthcare professionals to foster consumer awareness initiatives designed to empower individuals in making more informed health decisions.

One of the key objectives of consumer protection campaigns is to educate the public about the potential dangers associated with unverified health claims. Apricot seeds, once lauded for their supposed cancer-fighting properties due to their amygdalin content, pose significant health risks, including cyanide poisoning. Therefore, awareness campaigns are vital in disseminating factual information about the risks associated with their consumption. Initiatives might include distributing educational materials, hosting community workshops, or launching online campaigns to ensure that information about apricot seeds is readily accessible to those seeking guidance.

A critical component of effective consumer protection lies in empowering individuals with the skills necessary to evaluate health claims critically. This empowerment includes teaching the public how to differentiate between anecdotal evidence and scientifically substantiated claims. Campaigns can leverage various platforms, such as social media, to create engaging content that instructs individuals on how to assess the credibility of sources, spot red flags in health advertising, and recognize misleading claims. For instance, promoting the importance of scrutinizing the credentials of those making health assertions, the context of products in question, and the existence of empirical studies to support claims can significantly reduce the influence of misinformation.

These campaigns must also underscore the importance of seeking second opinions, particularly in the context of serious health issues like cancer treatment. Encouraging individuals to consult multiple healthcare professionals before adopting alternative treatments—especially those with little scientific endorsement—can prevent misguided choices. Healthcare professionals should be trained to communicate openly about alternatives while emphasizing the benefits of evidence-based medicine to inspire patient trust and collaboration.

Moreover, the role of advocates in protecting consumer rights is crucial. Health influencers and advocates must operate ethically and responsibly, particularly those with significant digital platforms, where their messages can reach vast audiences quickly. They should prioritize accuracy, transparency, and health literacy in their communications and steer clear of promoting remedies that lack scientific backing, such as apricot seeds for cancer.

As part of broader public health initiatives, awareness campaigns should also collaborate with regulatory bodies to ensure that messaging is aligned with consumer protection laws. These collaborations can amplify the reach of campaigns and provide additional authority to the messages disseminated. For example, sharing content backed by data and insights from reputable organizations like the FDA can foster public trust and enhance the legitimacy of health claims being contested.

Furthermore, leveraging technology and innovative communication strategies can help bolster consumer awareness. As health information is frequently sought online, campaigns must utilize digital tools effectively to educate users about the nature of valid health information. Strategies may include using social media platforms to create viral content that demystifies claims about apricot seeds and other remedies, producing infographics, or even developing mobile applications that provide users with vetted health resources.

Ultimately, consumer protection and awareness campaigns must engage various stakeholders, including healthcare professionals, community leaders, policymakers, and the medical community, to create a holistic approach to health education. Each group can contribute unique perspectives, resources, and expertise, furthering the mission to combat misinformation and empower consumers to make informed decisions about their health.

Consumer advocacy efforts can have profound impacts, ultimately leading to a more well-informed public capable of making decisions grounded in critical thinking and supported by scientific evidence. Through sustained collaboration, educational initiatives, and the prioritization of ethical health communication, advocates can help ensure that individuals navigate their health journeys more safely and confidently, significantly reducing the potential harms associated with unregulated alternative treatments like apricot seeds. As we move forward, fostering an environment where health information is scrutinized and validated will form the bedrock of consumer protection and awareness campaigns, leading to better health outcomes for all.

7.5. The Road Ahead: Legislation and Health Freedom

Legislation and health freedom represent a pivotal intersection in the ongoing discourse surrounding alternative treatments and public health. As misinformation surrounding remedies like apricot seeds continues to proliferate, the role of legislation becomes increasingly significant in shaping the landscape of health advocacy. Navigating these intricate waters requires a multifaceted approach that encompasses regulatory oversight, consumer protection, and informed decision-making, all while honoring individual freedoms.

In recent years, there has been a marked increase in legislative efforts aimed at governing the sale and promotion of alternative health products. These efforts respond to the surge in interest regarding natural remedies and the corresponding risks associated with their consumption—most notably evident in the controversy surrounding apricot seeds and their potent cyanide content. Regulatory bodies like the Food and Drug Administration (FDA) have issued guidelines aimed at protecting consumers from misleading claims while promoting safe practices.

The challenge lies in striking a balance between protecting public health and preserving health freedom—an essential principle that underscores an individual's right to make informed choices about their well-being. The concept of health freedom is foundational to many alternative medicine advocates, who argue that individuals should have the autonomy to seek out and choose treatments based on personal beliefs and experiences. This desire for health freedom is often fueled by a skepticism of established medical practices and the belief that natural remedies may offer safer alternatives.

However, unregulated health freedom can have unintended consequences, particularly when consumers are misled by unverified claims. Legislative frameworks must, therefore, navigate the delicate balance of ensuring consumer protection while respecting individual autonomy. Recent legislation has brought attention to this balancing act, emphasizing the need for transparency in marketing claims and heightened accountability for those promoting natural remedies that lack scientific support.

At the heart of this ongoing tension is the issue of misinformation. The dynamic landscape of health information—exacerbated by social media and digital platforms—enables rapid dissemination of both accurate and misleading health messages. The legislative response seeks to combat this misinformation by emphasizing the importance of consumer education and awareness campaigns. By equipping individuals with the tools needed to discern credible health claims from misleading ones, policymakers strive to foster an informed public capable of making wise health choices.

As legislative initiatives gain momentum, the role of health advocacy organizations becomes paramount. These groups rally to promote consumer rights and facilitate conversations around health choices that prioritize safety, efficacy, and evidence-based practices. Advocacy for informed health decisions often includes campaigns calling for stricter regulations on alternative treatments, such as apricot seeds. Such initiatives aim to instill confidence in consumers by ensuring that the products they encounter are subjected to rigorous safety evaluations.

Advocates for health freedom also play a crucial role in shaping public discourse around potential legislative measures. They maintain that a patient-centered approach to health necessitates a strong focus on individual choice while ensuring that harmful misinformation is effectively curbed. These discussions often prompt calls for collaborative efforts between legislators, health professionals, and consumer advocacy groups to develop comprehensive policies that reflect the diverse needs and values of society.

Legislation centered on health freedom should also prioritize inclusivity, recognizing that different communities may have varying beliefs surrounding health and wellness. Culturally sensitive approaches can foster trust and cooperation between public health initiatives and diverse populations, enhancing efforts to convey accurate information while respecting traditional beliefs. These dialogues serve as a testament to the importance of understanding individual contexts and experiences within the broader framework of health policy.

Looking ahead, the prospect of shaping health policy through responsible legislation represents both an opportunity and a challenge. As more individuals opt for alternative remedies like apricot seeds in their health regimens—driven by desires for natural solutions, empowerment, or even skepticism towards conventional medicine —the legal frameworks within which these choices reside must continue to adapt. Robust consumer education, regulatory oversight, and proactive collaboration among stakeholders are essential components in forging a future where health freedom and public safety coexist harmoniously.

Ultimately, the conversation surrounding legislation and health freedom must remain dynamic, responsive, and rooted in collaboration. As society grapples with evolving health narratives, the guiding principle should center on informed decision-making—one that empowers individuals to navigate their health choices responsibly while being safeguarded by the tenets of scientific evidence. By cultivating a holistic approach to health policy, communities can champion the pursuit of wellness that respects both individual rights and collective public health imperatives. It is through a commitment to informed decision-making, guided by legislative frameworks and empowered by health literacy, that individuals can advance their well-being and foster a society dedicated to lifelong wellness.

8. Consumer Awareness: Making Informed Health Choices

8.1. Navigating Health Information Online

Navigating health information online can be a daunting journey, especially in an age characterized by the rapid dissemination of information and the overwhelming number of sources available at our fingertips. As individuals increasingly turn to the internet for medical advice, the process of sifting through vast amounts of content to discern fact from fiction has become paramount. This subchapter aims to equip readers with the tools necessary for competent navigation through the complex digital health landscape, emphasizing critical thinking, skepticism, and reliable information sources.

The internet serves as both a blessing and a curse in accessing health information. On one hand, it has democratized knowledge, allowing individuals to seek guidance outside traditional healthcare settings. Social media, blogs, online forums, and health websites provide platforms for sharing experiences and fostering community support, which can be invaluable for those grappling with health challenges. However, this democratization also comes with considerable risks. The potential for the spread of misinformation is high, leading to harmful consequences if individuals take health claims at face value without careful analysis and validation.

To navigate health information online effectively, one must start by evaluating the credibility of sources. A critical approach begins with questioning the origin of the information, the qualifications of the authors, and the objectivity of the content. Health information from well-established, reputable organizations—such as the World Health Organization (WHO), the Centers for Disease Control and Prevention (CDC), or academic medical centers—should be prioritized, as these entities adhere to rigorous standards of research and evidence-based information. In contrast, content from unknown bloggers or social media influencers may not possess the same level of accuracy and reliability. Fact-checking websites can also serve as valuable reference points for validating claims.

The allure of personal stories can lead individuals astray as well, and caution is warranted when considering testimonials and anecdotal evidence. While such accounts can provide insight and a sense of community, they do not replace the need for empirical evidence. Positive experiences shared by individuals should not be misconstrued as definitive proof of efficacy, especially for treatments lacking scientific validation. For instance, the narrative surrounding apricot seeds as a potential cancer cure often rests on vivid personal stories, overshadowing the scientific consensus that emphasizes the risk of cyanide poisoning associated with their consumption.

In addition to examining the source, spotting red flags in health advice is crucial for discerning reliable information from unfounded claims. Claims that promise quick fixes, miraculous results, or overly simplistic solutions to complex health issues are often indicative of misleading or untrustworthy content. Phrases such as "miracle cure," "secret remedy," or "guaranteed results" should raise immediate skepticism. Furthermore, any health advice that emphasizes fear, desperation, or urgency often serves to manipulate individuals into making hasty decisions, as seen in the promotion of apricot seeds. The framing of health choices should always be balanced, emphasizing both benefits and risks.

The importance of second opinions cannot be overstated when making health decisions based on online information. Consulting multiple healthcare professionals or cross-referencing different sources can lead to a more well-rounded understanding of any health issue. Engaging with healthcare providers who can contextualize information based on individual circumstances is vital, especially when considering alternative treatments. This dialogue empowers individuals with knowledge while protecting them from potential pitfalls associated with self-diagnosis or reliance on unverified remedies.

Empowering patients should be the overarching goal of navigating health information online. Public health initiatives can play a significant role in fostering health literacy, teaching individuals how to evaluate health claims critically, and providing straightforward, actionable steps for finding reliable content. Community-focused workshops, educational webinars, and engaging resources can demystify health information while nurturing a culture of inquiry and skepticism. Building knowledge and awareness should be continuous endeavors, ensuring that individuals are equipped with the tools needed to discern evidence from hearsay throughout their health journeys.

Ultimately, the capacity to navigate health information online successfully is an essential skill in today's information-driven world. Individual responsibility toward informed health choices can help mitigate the risks posed by misinformation and promote well-being. By grounding health decisions in credible sources, maintaining a critical eye toward claims, and fostering open communication with healthcare professionals, individuals can navigate their paths to wellness with confidence and clarity. Embracing this proactive approach to health information empowers individuals not only to embrace the benefits of the system but also to challenge misinformation—leading to more informed and safer health choices.

8.2. Evaluating Claims with a Critical Eye

In evaluating health claims with a critical eye, it is essential to approach information with skepticism and a methodical mindset. The prevalence of health misinformation, particularly in the realm of alternative treatments such as apricot seeds for cancer, necessitates that individuals engage in a rigorous analysis of the claims presented to them. This critical evaluation covers several pivotal components, beginning with the source of information and extending to the evidence supporting specific claims.

Start by examining the origin of the information. Reputable sources —such as governmental health organizations (e.g., the CDC, WHO), peer-reviewed scientific journals, or accredited health institutions—

should take precedence over anecdotal accounts or personal testimonials. Misinformation often arises in spaces that lack oversight, such as social media platforms and alternative health websites, which can promote unverified claims without scientific backing. By prioritizing information from established health authorities, individuals are more likely to engage with content that has undergone thorough scrutiny and evaluation.

Moreover, it is crucial to question the qualifications of the authors presenting the information. Consider whether they have the necessary expertise in the relevant field, including credentials and a history of credible contributions to health discussions. An individual without qualifications, presenting health information as fact, may not fully understand the complexities of medicine or the potential risks associated with unverified claims, such as the consumption of apricot seeds.

In addition to scrutinizing the source, evaluate the quality of the evidence presented. Claims should ideally be backed by empirical research—particularly large-scale clinical trials or systematic reviews —demonstrating efficacy and safety for the treatment in question. Phases of research typically follow a meticulous process: preclinical studies are conducted, followed by clinical trials that may go through several phases before receiving regulatory approval. A lack of substantial evidence or reliance solely on personal anecdotes should color the reader's interpretation of the information. For example, while some individuals may share success stories regarding apricot seed consumption, these personal experiences cannot substitute for scientific validation regarding treatment effectiveness or safety.

Attention to potential conflicts of interest is another critical aspect of evaluating health claims. Investigate whether the author or promoter of the treatment stands to gain financially from the sale of a product that lacks proven benefits. Often, proponents of alternative treatments have a vested interest in promoting their claims, resulting in biased information. Understanding the motivations behind specific claims can help individuals navigate the murky waters of health misinformation.

Furthermore, understanding the balance between risk and benefit is vital when evaluating health claims. Any pill, supplement, or natural remedy has the potential for side effects or adverse reactions. For example, while apricot seeds are marketed for their purported cancer-fighting properties, the significant risk of cyanide toxicity must be a priority in discussions surrounding their use. Engaging with the nuances of risk assessment allows individuals to make informed decisions by weighing the potential benefits against the possible dangers.

It is also essential to be aware of cognitive biases that may affect decision-making processes. Many individuals fall victim to confirmation bias—favoring information that aligns with their existing beliefs while ignoring evidence to the contrary. Striving for objectivity requires remaining open to new information, allowing for revisions in beliefs as new evidence emerges. This critical mindset encourages a holistic understanding of health claims, reducing the susceptibility to misinformation.

The discourse surrounding apricot seeds and their purported cancer-curing properties exemplifies the importance of a critical evaluation of claims. Despite their promotion by various advocates as a magical remedy, the overwhelming body of scientific literature is at odds with these assertions, highlighting significant risks without substantiated benefits. Encouragingly, members of the scientific community continue to promote awareness and education, fostering a culture that values inquiry, transparency, and informed decision-making.

In conclusion, evaluating claims with a critical eye is not merely a useful skill—it's an essential practice in navigating the ever-evolving landscape of health information. By approaching health claims in a rigorous, discerning manner, individuals can better safeguard their wellness decisions against the pitfalls of misinformation, ultimately empowering them to make choices grounded in safety and efficacy.

8.3. Spotting Red Flags in Health Advice

Spotting red flags in health advice requires a discerning eye, especially in an era where misinformation can spread rapidly through digital platforms. Health claims, especially those pertaining to alternative treatments such as apricot seeds, should be scrutinized to separate harmful myths from credible information. A reflective stance on health suggestions can prevent individuals from making misguided decisions that may jeopardize their well-being. It's essential to be aware of specific indicators that signal a need for caution.

One prominent red flag is the use of sensationalized language and promises of miraculous cures. Claims that a product can "cure" a severe illness like cancer in a short period should be met with skepticism. These statements often appeal to emotions rather than facts and can lead to dangerous choices, particularly when accompanied by urgent messaging that triggers fear or despair in individuals facing health crises. More grounded health advice will typically emphasize balanced treatment approaches, highlighting the complexity of diseases and acknowledging that no single remedy can address all health issues.

It's also important to question the qualifications of those making the claims. If the person promoting a remedy lacks relevant training or expertise—whether in medicine, nutrition, or pharmacology—this raises the question of the credibility of the advice. Health influencers or advocates without professional backgrounds in scientific fields frequently rely on anecdotal evidence rather than evidence-based research, which can lead to the propagation of misleading narratives. Engaging with information produced by recognized experts or organizations in the field will generally yield more reliable insights.

Another red flag is a lack of transparency regarding scientific evidence supporting the claims. If the advice does not reference empirical studies, credible clinical trials, or established research published in reputable medical journals, its validity is called into question. Trustworthy health information will often cite scientific studies and provide a rationale for the claims being made, whereas flawed advice may dismiss the need for evidence altogether. This is particularly relevant in discussions about apricot seeds for cancer treatment, where the absence of scientific backing for the supposed benefits should evoke caution.

The promotion of alternative treatments often includes testimonials that advocate for products like apricot seeds. While personal stories can offer insights into individual experiences, they cannot substitute for scientific evidence. Relying solely on testimonials creates a bias known as confirmation bias, where only positive experiences are amplified while negative outcomes are ignored or downplayed. This underscores the importance of considering a broader range of experiences and carefully weighing anecdotal evidence against established research.

Additionally, the allure of a natural remedy can distort critical thinking. The belief that anything derived from nature is inherently safe can lead individuals to overlook potentially harmful side effects. For apricot seeds, despite being natural, the presence of cyanogenic compounds that can lead to poisoning is a significant risk that must not be underestimated. Claims promoting the seeds without addressing these dangers exemplify a failure to provide balanced information, signaling that caution is warranted.

Price points and the marketing strategies accompanying health products also merit scrutiny. When products are marketed with exorbitant prices or packaged as exclusive solutions to dire health problems, red flags should be raised. These tactics often exploit the vulnerabilities of consumers who are searching for solutions in their health journeys, preying on their hopes and fears.

To effectively spot these red flags, individuals must cultivate a critical mindset. Engaging in health literacy—developing the skills to assess and evaluate health information—is particularly important in this digital age, where misinformation proliferates. By arming oneself with the tools to critically analyze health claims, individuals can be proactive rather than reactive when faced with emerging narratives surrounding alternative treatments.

Moreover, discussing health choices with healthcare professionals can offer valuable insight and guidance. Providers can validate or refute claims based on scientific research while offering alternative recommendations that are both safe and effective. Such dialogues foster a collaborative environment where informed choices can be made, ensuring that individuals retain a sense of agency in their health decisions.

In summary, recognizing red flags in health advice is a critical skill in an era rife with misinformation. By remaining vigilant and employing critical thinking, individuals can navigate the complex landscape of health information successfully, making choices grounded in evidence rather than appealing but potentially harmful narratives. Such discernment is especially crucial when considering remedies such as apricot seeds, where the risks associated with their consumption must always overshadow unverified claims of efficacy.

8.4. The Importance of Second Opinions

The discourse surrounding health decisions is often fraught with complexities and uncertainties, particularly in the context of serious illnesses such as cancer. Among these complexities lies a critical, yet frequently overlooked, aspect of medical decision-making: the importance of second opinions. In a landscape characterized by a growing interest in alternative treatments, like apricot seeds as purported cancer cures, the role of seeking a second opinion becomes paramount in ensuring informed, safe, and effective health choices.

One primary rationale for obtaining a second opinion is the inherent variability in medical opinions and treatment recommendations. The pathway to cancer diagnosis and treatment can be fraught with emotional strain and significant life-altering choices. Each healthcare provider may possess a unique perspective shaped by their education, experience, and practice style. While one oncologist may advocate for aggressive treatment measures, another may suggest a more conservative approach, possibly integrating alternative therapies. Such differences underscore the necessity of exploring diverse viewpoints to facilitate an informed decision-making process that aligns with the patient's individual values and circumstances.

Moreover, the potential pitfalls of misdiagnosis highlight the need for corroboration in medical advice. Cancer diagnostics can be highly complex, often necessitating a range of tests, imaging, and specialized evaluations. A second opinion can serve as a valuable check against erroneous diagnoses or confusion regarding the appropriate course of treatment. When patients seek additional validation from another expert, they are more likely to feel confidence in the treatment plan, whether it involves traditional therapies, complementary approaches, or even the avoidance of risky alternatives like apricot seeds.

There is an inherent value in peer collaboration and remapping the treatment landscape for each patient. Obtaining a second opinion often opens doors to collaborative discussions that extend beyond a singular clinician's view. When connecting with multiple specialists, patients can benefit from a synthesis of knowledge that reflects a broader array of expertise, potentially highlighting innovative treatment options that may have otherwise been overlooked.

Consider the case of a patient diagnosed with cancer who is drawn to the narrative surrounding apricot seeds as a natural cure. They may experience initial enthusiasm when encountering testimonials of others who claim success due to these seeds. However, before committing to this alternative solution, consulting with an additional oncologist could unveil critical insights about the scientific consensus surrounding apricot seeds and their inherent risks, particularly regarding cyanide toxicity linked to amygdalin. A second opinion allows the patient to weigh anecdotal evidence against empirical data, enabling more informed decision-making regarding their health.

Emotional factors also play a substantial role in the decision to pursue a second opinion. Patients may enter treatment discussions with preconceived notions and emotional biases that can cloud rational judgment. Seeking a second opinion can alleviate feelings of anxiety, uncertainty, and doubt, allowing patients to navigate their health journeys with greater assurance. The act of obtaining an additional viewpoint signifies proactive engagement with one's health and fosters a sense of empowerment, which is particularly crucial in the face of life-altering diagnoses.

In addition, the broader ethical implications of second opinions must be considered. Patients have the right to fully understand their diagnosis, treatment options, and the risks involved. Engaging with multiple healthcare providers fosters transparency and informed consent—elements deeply entrenched within ethical medical practice. It ensures that patients are equipped to make choices derived from comprehensive information, combining perspectives from various experts that respect the complexities of their individual health circumstances.

While time constraints and healthcare access can pose challenges in seeking multiple opinions, the long-term benefits of vigilance and scrutiny far outweigh the momentary inconvenience. Efforts to facilitate second opinions through health education campaigns must take precedence, empowering patients to advocate for their health with confidence. Inclusion of second opinion policies in healthcare systems can further normalize the practice, encouraging dialogue that reinforces patient autonomy.

In an age where misinformation about alternative treatments can readily proliferate, the importance of second opinions emerges as a beacon of critical thinking and scientific inquiry. Individual agency should always extend to evaluating health information and consulting multiple experts, particularly in the context of significant health crises like cancer. As narratives around treatments like apricot seeds continue to captivate the public imagination, the significance of second opinions will only grow, championing informed decision-making and ultimately fostering safer, more effective health choices.

In conclusion, seeking a second opinion stands as a cornerstone of responsible health management. It empowers individuals to navigate the complexities of their diagnoses and treatment paths while ensuring that decisions are rooted in a comprehensive understanding of their health condition. As we strive to counteract the allure of over-simplified solutions and the risks associated with alternative claims, the practice of securing second opinions must remain an essential avenue for advocacy, safety, and individualized care.

8.5. Empowering Patients: Advocating for Your Health

Empowering patients in their health advocacy journey is of paramount importance, especially in an era where misinformation about treatments can be dangerously alluring. The notion that individuals can take control of their health decisions resonates strongly in a society increasingly skeptical of conventional medicine. This empowerment not only involves making informed choices but also advocating for oneself within the healthcare system. As patients become more proactive in their health management, they must also recognize the power and responsibility that come with seeking accurate information and accountability in their health choices.

One of the first steps in empowering patients is fostering health literacy. Understanding medical terminology, treatment options, and the implications of various approaches equips individuals to engage meaningfully with healthcare professionals. Health literacy branches beyond reading pamphlets; it encompasses the ability to interpret health information critically, distinguishing between credible medical sources and anecdotal claims. In navigating discussions about alternative treatments, such as apricot seeds for cancer, a well-informed patient can ask pertinent questions, weigh risks, and make decisions aligned with established medical guidelines.

Encouraging collaboration and open communication between patients and healthcare providers is another pivotal aspect of empowerment. Patients should feel comfortable discussing their preferences, concerns, and desires for alternative therapies. This dialogue can lead to more tailored treatment plans that respect individual choices while simultaneously adhering to medical evidence. Empowered patients are typically more engaged in their care, fostering a partnership that supports shared decision-making without compromising safety.

Advocacy can take many forms—from engaging in conversations about treatment options to joining support groups that foster discussion around health experiences. Patients can also become advocates for health policy, pushing for regulations that prioritize safety, transparency, and the welfare of individuals. Engaging with advocacy organizations can empower patients to amplify their voices on issues affecting healthcare access, quality, and education about alternative treatments.

Moreover, patients can harness the power of community—both online and offline—as they seek information, support, and shared experiences. The internet provides platforms for connection, although caution is needed when engaging with unverified information. By connecting with others who share similar health challenges, patients can gain insights into how others navigate their choices, bolstering confidence in their own advocacy efforts. However, this community should also emphasize critical thinking and evidence-based discussions to counter the spread of misinformation.

It is important to address the emotional landscape that patients traverse in their health journeys. Especially when facing serious conditions like cancer, the psychological toll can lead individuals to seek out comforting solutions, sometimes leading them toward unproven treatments. Patients must recognize the complex interplay between hope, fear, and health decision-making. Empowering patients involves not only the dissemination of information but also support in processing emotional factors that impact choices. Mental health support can complement physical health management, helping individuals navigate their treatment journeys more effectively.

Finally, advocacy extends beyond the individual to interactions with public health policy. Patients can engage in campaigns demanding more stringent regulations on alternative treatments that lack scientific backing, such as apricot seeds. This not only protects individuals from potential harm but also reflects a collective commitment to safer health choices. By participating in advocacy efforts, patients can help create an environment where the promotion of alternative remedies is informed by rigorous scientific evaluation rather than fallacious claims.

In conclusion, empowering patients to advocate for their health encompasses a multifaceted approach that includes cultivating health literacy, fostering open communication with healthcare providers, and building supportive communities. As individual advocates, patients are urged to engage actively with their healthcare discussions, balancing the personal dimensions of their health journeys with critical evaluation of the information they encounter. By doing so, they can not only make informed health choices but also contribute to a larger movement towards a healthcare landscape grounded in safety, science, and informed decision-making.

9. How Misinformation Propagates

9.1. The Role of Social Media

In the contemporary landscape of health and wellness, social media has emerged as a double-edged sword, wielding both the promise of accessibility and the peril of misinformation. With the rise of platforms such as Facebook, Instagram, Twitter, and TikTok, individuals have unprecedented access to health information and personal stories that can profoundly influence perceptions of various treatments, especially alternative remedies like apricot seeds. The role of social media in shaping the discourse around health not only encompasses the potential for positive outreach but also the pressing challenges posed by the propagation of dangerous myths.

The allure of social media lies in its ability to connect people and facilitate the swift dissemination of information. This capability promotes community building among individuals who may feel isolated in their health journeys, allowing them to share experiences, resources, and firsthand accounts of various treatments. For example, individuals grappling with cancer may seek solidarity from those who tout "natural" solutions, such as apricot seeds, leading to a viral trend that amplifies these narratives. The sharing of personal testimonials can create a compelling and emotional narrative, often overshadowing scientific evidence or cautionary advice from healthcare professionals.

However, this viral nature makes social media platforms fertile ground for misinformation and pseudoscience. Claims surrounding the purported efficacy of apricot seeds as a cancer cure are often presented without adequate scientific backing, relying instead on sensationalized anecdotes. The sheer volume of content generated by health influencers, combined with the algorithms that prioritize engagement, can lead to the elevation of anecdotes over facts. Testimonials describing miraculous recoveries become viral sensations, easily convincing others to adopt unproven treatments, even when these narratives neglect to mention significant risks—like cyanide poisoning associated with apricot seed consumption.

Recent studies reveal that emotional resonance often supersedes logical reasoning when individuals engage with health-related content online. The psychology behind liking, sharing, or saving posts that promote the idea of natural remedies draws on an innate desire for hope and simplicity—two powerful emotions that can override skepticism or critical thinking. As a result, users may unconsciously dismiss scientific evidence contradicting these claims, focusing instead on the persuasive power of shared stories and personal successes.

Compounding this issue is the challenge of misinformation. A multitude of voices and perspectives flood social media, making it challenging for users to discern credible sources from dubious claims. The rapid cycle of information means that incorrect, misleading, or exaggerated health advice can spread quickly, as sensational content gains traction and is further propagated through likes and shares. This phenomenon illustrates the need for health professionals and organizations to engage strategically on social media platforms, crafting clear, concise, and accurate messages that can counteract the allure of sensationalized health claims.

Efforts to tackle misinformation must begin with improving health literacy at both individual and community levels. Public health officials can use social media as a tool to disseminate accurate information about cancer prevention and treatment and to debunk common myths, including those surrounding apricot seeds. Collaborative campaigns involving healthcare professionals, trusted influencers, and regulatory agencies can help amplify credible messages and reach more extensive audiences.

Creating partnerships with social media platforms to identify and limit the proliferation of false health information is another crucial step. Flagging a misleading post or redirecting users to reputable sources can significantly impact the spread of misinformation, promoting awareness and informed choices among users. Initiatives geared toward verifying health-related content and offering prompts to seek professional advice can empower individuals to reflect critically on the health information they encounter.

Ultimately, while social media offers a powerful channel through which health narratives unfold, it also presents considerable challenges that demand vigilant scrutiny. Individuals navigating health information online must cultivate a critical mindset, guiding their engagement with content based on evidence rather than anecdote. The quest for health knowledge is fraught with complexities, but confronting misinformation requires a collaborative effort—a united front of healthcare professionals, influencers, and consumers committed to prioritizing accuracy, safety, and evidence-based practices in health discourse.

In conclusion, the role of social media in health discussions embodies both opportunity and challenge. It is essential to harness its potential to connect and inform while vigilantly confronting and dispelling harmful myths. As we continue this digital dialogue surrounding health, let's cultivate an informed community dedicated to making wise, evidence-based choices in pursuit of wellness.

9.2. Viral Trends and Their Impact on Health

As we delve into the phenomenon of viral trends and their impact on health, we embark on a journey that scrutinizes the intricate relationship between the dispersion of health-related narratives and the consequences that ensue. Viral trends can engulf social media platforms, evoke powerful emotions, and, often, mislead individuals into unverified and potentially hazardous health practices. This dynamic is especially poignant in the realm of alternative treatments, where stories of natural remedies like apricot seeds—celebrated by some as miraculous cancer cures—captivate the public imagination and often inadvertently jeopardize health decisions.

The digital age has transformed the way health information is disseminated, with viral trends becoming a prominent facet of consumer health engagement. When a purported remedy, such as apricot seeds, catches the collective consciousness of social media users, it can lead to rapid proliferation of anecdotes and testimonials, all of which can amplify their perceived legitimacy. Personal stories—a powerful medium for establishing emotional connections—often dominate these narratives, encouraging individuals to embrace solutions that resonate with their desires for simplicity and hope in health challenges.

However, this emotional response can obscure the underlying truths about such treatments. The compelling nature of viral health claims often overshadows critical analyses of safety, efficacy, and scientific validity. For example, while some individuals may share accounts of positive experiences with apricot seeds, they frequently neglect to include the significant risks associated with their use, namely the potential for cyanide poisoning. This selective sharing cultivates an environment where anecdotal evidence is celebrated, but contrasting scientific research is downplayed or dismissed.

The implications are profound, as viral trends can divert individuals from evidence-based treatments, leading to dire consequences. The public's embrace of apricot seeds as a hopeful alternative to conventional therapies illustrates the risk of relying on trends that can encourage spontaneous and uncritical acceptance of health claims without due diligence. When health narratives foster a belief in simple solutions to complex health crises, the urge to forego established medical practices can inadvertently arise, culminating in detrimental health outcomes.

Moreover, the speed at which information is circulated on social media complicates efforts to impose regulatory checks on misleading health claims. The rapid-fire nature of viral trends makes it challenging for regulatory bodies and health authorities to respond effectively, often resulting in difficulties countering prevailing narratives before they embed themselves in popular consciousness. This highlights the urgent need for proactive consumer education initiatives that can capture audience attention swiftly and disseminate counter-narratives grounded in scientific rigor.

Addressing viral trends and their implications requires coordinated efforts from multiple stakeholders, including healthcare professionals, public health officials, and advocates for health literacy. Digital health communication strategies must be developed with an emphasis on credibility, clarity, and proactive engagement with the community. By harnessing digital platforms, health organizations can craft messages that not only educate but also resonate emotionally with their audiences, blurring the line between information and engagement while reframing the dialogue surrounding unverified remedies.

As we delve deeper into the specifics of viral trends, the essential role of health advocates and influencers in shaping the narrative becomes apparent. With significant reach and impact, these individuals can serve as champions for accurate information, amplifying scientifically sound messages that prioritize safety and efficacy. It is incumbent upon them to utilize trusted sources and present findings that reflect the current scientific consensus, steering their audiences away from harmful misinformation.

In conclusion, the power of viral trends and their impact on health encapsulates a complex interplay of narrative, emotion, and information-sharing in the digital age. While these trends can foster connections and serve as platforms for discourse, they also pose significant risks when they drive individuals toward unverified remedies like apricot seeds. As we maneuver through this intricate landscape, the necessity for critical engagement, responsible advocacy, and dissemination of scientifically validated information becomes ever more apparent. Navigating the realm of health information requires not only an understanding of the allure of viral trends but also a commitment to building a culture of informed decision-making that champions safety, efficacy, and overall well-being.

9.3. The Power of Personal Testimonials

The impact of personal testimonials in health discussions is profound, especially when intertwined with topics as contentious as apricot seeds' role in cancer treatment. These narratives, often rife with emotional weight and persuasive power, can shape perceptions and influence decision-making in ways that scientific evidence struggles to match. The allure of personal stories—those accounts of miraculous recoveries, anecdotal successes, and transformative experiences—often leads individuals to favor personal anecdotes over empirical data. This tendency poses significant challenges for public health, as emotional resonance, rather than scientific scrutiny, frequently guides choices regarding health interventions.

Examining the phenomenon of personal testimonials in the realm of health reveals a compelling duality: they function as both powerful agents of change and potential conduits for misinformation. On the one hand, personal testimonials can humanize health challenges, making complex medical conditions more relatable. They evoke empathy and create narratives that resonate deeply with individuals facing similar struggles, providing a sense of connection and community. For many seeking alternative cures, like apricot seeds, these stories can offer comfort, hope, and the belief that a simple solution exists to combat a formidable adversary like cancer.

The perils of relying on testimonials, however, become evident when examining cases where outcomes are presented without context. Often, the success stories surrounding apricot seeds gloss over the critical scientific realities associated with their consumption. While an individual may share a tale of improvement after consuming apricot seeds, such accounts may lack transparency regarding possible adverse effects, including the risks of cyanide poisoning from amygdalin, which can lead to severe health complications. This lack of comprehensive information can foster misguided beliefs that apricot seeds are a safe and effective remedy, potentially leading others to forgo evidence-based treatments in favor of unverified claims.

The role of personal testimonials becomes even more pronounced amid the rise of social media, where emotional narratives can quickly gain traction and achieve viral status. Shared experiences often find fertile ground among communities seeking support, driving the popularity of alternative health remedies. A single viral post about the efficacy of apricot seeds can generate significant discussions, wherein testimonials proliferate and reinforce a shared belief in the remedy's power. This cycle perpetuates a narrative that prioritizes anecdotal evidence, ultimately drowning out critical voices emphasizing the need for empirical validation.

Such dynamics showcase the need for healthcare professionals to engage critically with personal testimony while promoting evidence-based practices. While it is essential to validate the experiences of individuals, skilled communication strategies can guide conversations toward a balanced understanding of the risks and benefits associated with various health interventions. This entails fostering dialogues that explore the nuances of health decision-making—encouraging individuals to weigh personal experiences alongside robust scientific inquiries.

Navigating the intricate landscape shaped by personal testimonials requires the establishment of guidelines around health communication. Advocacy organizations, healthcare providers, and public health officials can work collaboratively to create an environment that values both lived experiences and scientific evidence. This might involve developing public health campaigns that emphasize the importance of informed decision-making, encouraging individuals to seek accurate information, and foster critical engagement with personal stories.

In essence, while personal testimonials have the power to inspire and connect, caution must be exercised in portraying claims as indisputable validation of efficacy. By redirecting the focus toward collaborative health advocacy that harmonizes personal narratives with scientific understanding, individuals can navigate their health choices more effectively. Cultivating an environment wherein emotional resonance coexists harmoniously with empirical scrutiny ultimately promotes wiser health decisions, ensuring that hope remains grounded in safety, efficacy, and informed choice.

Moreover, embracing the complexity of testimonials means recognizing the potential consequences of misleading narratives. As such, creating channels for counter-testimonials—stories of those who have faced adverse reactions or who emphasize the importance of evidence-based medicine—can offer a more rounded perspective. Encouraging open conversations about the limitations of personal experiences in the medical realm creates space for critical reflection and informed discourse, paving the way for wiser health choices that are both compassionate and grounded in science.

Lastly, personal testimonials are not inherently detrimental; rather, they can serve as valuable teaching moments. By fostering a culture that encourages individuals to share their experiences while simultaneously embedding discussions about scientific principles and safety, we can transform anecdotes into tools for empowerment. Personal stories, when contextualized within sound medical guidance, can enhance community engagement in health, bridging the gap between lived experience and scientific inquiry. Such an integrative approach not only honors individual narratives but also upholds the commitment to informed, evidence-based health practices—a harmonious balance that ultimately supports the wellness of individuals within the larger community.

9.4. Tackling Pseudoscience in the Modern Age

In the age of increasing accessibility to information through the web, the proliferation of pseudoscientific claims poses a significant challenge to critical thinking and informed decision-making. Misinformation regarding health practices, particularly regarding controversial topics such as apricot seeds as potential cancer treatments, has become alarmingly prevalent. As individuals grapple with the allure of simplistic solutions to complex health crises, the responsibility to tackle pseudoscience falls on various stakeholders, from individuals to policymakers.

One primary avenue for confronting these challenges is through education. As individuals navigate the vast sea of health information, they must be equipped with the skills necessary to discern credible research from dubious claims. Public health initiatives must prioritize health literacy, fostering the capability to evaluate sources critically, understand research methodologies, and seek corroborating evidence before adopting any health practices. This initiative can manifest in community workshops, online courses, or social media campaigns that promote evidence-based approaches to health, emphasizing the importance of consulting healthcare professionals when making decisions related to health interventions.

In addition to individual responsibility, there is a pressing need for robust regulatory frameworks that address the rampant promotion of unverified health claims. Regulatory agencies must actively monitor and evaluate the sale and marketing of alternative treatments, ensuring that consumers are protected from misleading assertions. Governments should mandate clear labeling and evidence-backed claims for any health product marketed to the public, enforcing penalties for misleading marketing practices. Stricter regulations surrounding the dissemination of health information online could discourage the spread of unverified claims and promote a more informed public discourse.

Social media platforms play a significant role in the dissemination of misinformation. The algorithms that govern these platforms often favor sensational content, which can lead to the spread of pseudo-sciences like those surrounding apricot seeds. Social media companies must take on greater accountability by implementing measures that prioritize verified health information, flagging content that lacks credible substantiation, and promoting health campaigns grounded in scientific evidence. Partnering with public health authorities could be instrumental in enhancing the quality of information circulating across these networks.

Another crucial component in tackling pseudoscience is leveraging the power of trusted voices—healthcare professionals, researchers, and public health advocates—to inject factual information into the ongoing conversations about health practices. By engaging in proactive outreach, these individuals can demystify health claims that lack scientific support and educate consumers on the risks associated with relying solely on alternative treatments. Public trust in healthcare professionals is paramount, and their active participation in discussions can help foster a more informed dialogue.

Moreover, understanding the emotional and psychological motivations driving individuals toward alternative remedies is essential in addressing misinformation effectively. Many people may turn to natural solutions like apricot seeds out of fear, desperation, or a desire for control over their health choices. Acknowledging these emotional factors in health communication can create opportunities for empathetic discussions, allowing healthcare advocates to address concerns while providing scientifically validated alternatives.

Pseudoscience thrives in an environment where information is oversimplified and devoid of nuance. The narratives surrounding natural remedies often paint a simplistic picture—the idea that a single substance can eradicate a complex illness. By promoting a more comprehensive understanding of health that acknowledges the multifaceted nature of diseases and the importance of evidence-based practices, we pave the way for informed discussions about treatment options. This shift in narrative requires not only the input of individuals but also a collective commitment to ethical health practices.

In conclusion, tackling pseudoscience in the modern age requires a multifaceted approach that combines individual responsibility, education, regulatory oversight, and collaboration with trusted health professionals. As we navigate an era overwhelmed by conflicting health information, fostering a culture of critical thinking and informed decision-making is paramount. By embracing these values and working together to counter misinformation, we can empower individuals to make wiser health choices that prioritize safety and efficacy, ultimately leading to a more informed, healthier society.

9.5. Ways to Stop the Spread of False Information

In the fight against the spread of false information, particularly regarding health claims and alternative treatments, it is essential to adopt a multifaceted approach that involves critical engagement, education, and collaboration among various stakeholders. The narrative surrounding apricot seeds—and their purported properties as a cancer cure—illustrates how easily misinformation can proliferate, often compelling individuals to make decisions based on hope rather than sound scientific principles. Here are several effective ways to address and curb the spread of false information:

One of the primary strategies involves enhancing public health literacy. By equipping individuals with the skills needed to discern credible health information from unverified claims, we empower them to make informed health choices. Educational campaigns can focus on teaching the public how to evaluate the credibility of health sources, the importance of looking for peer-reviewed studies, and the value of consulting healthcare professionals before adopting any new treatment. Interactive workshops, community seminars, and online courses can all serve as platforms for disseminating this knowledge.

Furthermore, it's crucial to promote critical thinking among the public when evaluating health information. This includes encouraging individuals to question the motivations behind health claims, particularly when they are presented without adequate evidence. An approach known as the "SIFT" method—Stop, Investigate, Find better coverage, and Trace claims—can guide users in verifying the reliability of information encountered online. By fostering a culture of skepticism, we can diminish the appeal of sensationalized health claims while promoting more thoughtful engagement with health narratives.

The role that technology plays in disseminating information cannot be overlooked. Social media platforms should be encouraged to enhance their policies surrounding health misinformation. This can involve implementing tools that flag or provide context for misleading claims and directing users to verified sources of information. Collaborative partnerships between tech companies and public health organizations can further serve to amplify accurate health messages, thereby reducing the visibility of harmful misinformation about treatments like apricot seeds.

Additionally, public health authorities and health professionals must actively engage in the conversation surrounding alternative treatments. By participating in discussions across digital platforms, they can provide context, challenge misleading claims, and offer evidence-based guidance. Taking a proactive stance in addressing misinformation can both inform the public and build trust in credible sources of information.

Another significant avenue for tackling false information is engaging with influential figures in health and wellness, including bloggers, social media influencers, and community leaders. Encouraging these figures to adopt responsible communication practices—by emphasizing scientific evidence, acknowledging risks, and prioritizing patient safety—can help mitigate the circulation of unverified claims. By using their platforms to relay accurate health information, these influencers can play an instrumental role in countering the narratives that promote harmful remedies.

Lastly, addressing the emotional and psychological factors that drive individuals toward alternative treatments is essential in combating misinformation. Understanding the context behind why individuals may search for natural remedies like apricot seeds—often driven by a desire for agency or dissatisfaction with conventional medicine—can inform how we approach health communication. By offering support, fostering open discussions about fears and concerns, and providing clear, honest information about health risks associated with unverified claims, we can create an environment conducive to informed decision-making.

In conclusion, combating the spread of false information, particularly regarding health claims surrounding alternatives like apricot seeds, requires a comprehensive approach that prioritizes education, critical engagement, and collaboration. By enhancing health literacy, promoting critical thinking, leveraging technology, engaging influential voices, and addressing the underlying emotional factors that drive individuals towards alternative remedies, we can work collectively to create a more informed public. In doing so, we not only empower individuals to make wise health choices but safeguard public health against the dangers of misinformation.

10. Ethical Considerations in Promoting Alternative Treatments

10.1. Responsibility of Health Influencers

The rise of health influencers has dramatically transformed the landscape of public health communication, particularly with respect to alternative treatments like apricot seeds for cancer. While these individuals often seek to share information and provide support to those navigating health challenges, the responsibility that comes with their influence cannot be overstated. In a realm where personal narratives and anecdotal evidence frequently capture the public's attention, influencers have the power to shape perceptions, motivate decisions, and potentially mislead their audiences—often without the oversight provided by scientific rigor.

Health influencers, operating in the digital age, rely on platforms where likes, shares, and follower counts dictate visibility. This can lead to a culture where sensational claims about natural remedies are favored over scientifically grounded information. The widespread belief that apricot seeds hold curative properties for serious ailments like cancer serves as a cautionary tale regarding the potential consequences of unchecked influence. Health influencers who promote such claims without acknowledging the risks associated with cyanide toxicity present in the seeds fail to fulfill their ethical obligation to provide balanced, evidence-based perspectives.

As individuals seeking health advice are often drawn to personal stories and shared experiences, influencers must recognize the ethical implications of their promotions. Authenticity and honesty should be the cornerstones of their communication strategies. This means being transparent about personal experiences and the uncertainties associated with alternative treatments. Influencers should demonstrate a commitment to presenting information that reflects a diversity of opinions and recognizes the importance of traditional medical practices alongside alternative approaches.

Moreover, the responsibility of health influencers extends to actively engaging with scientific research and public health guidelines. By collaborating with healthcare professionals and organizations, they can form a stronger foundation of credibility for their content. This partnership approach allows influencers to educate their audiences effectively while simultaneously advocating for safety and informed health choices. A commitment to research-backed evidence not only elevates the influencers' responsibility but also empowers consumers to make knowledgeable health decisions.

The ethical landscape also encompasses the consideration of potential conflicts of interest. As influencers may promote specific products or treatments for financial gain, transparency regarding partnerships and sponsored content becomes vital. Audiences should be able to distinguish between genuine endorsements based on health benefits and purely commercial motivations. By disclosing financial arrangements or affiliations, influencers can build trust with their followers while reinforcing their ethical accountability.

Critically, the responsibility of health influencers is not limited to promoting content; it includes actively countering misinformation —especially when it pertains to unverified claims about alternative treatments. Engaging in conversations about the limits of certain natural remedies while advocating for established medical practices will significantly deter the spread of harmful myths. By fostering dialogue around critical health issues, influencers can guide their followers toward more nuanced understandings of health options, empowering them to make informed choices anchored in safety and efficacy.

In summary, health influencers occupy a unique and powerful space in the discourse surrounding alternative treatments like apricot seeds. The responsibility they bear is both significant and multifaceted: it involves informing their audiences with integrity, advocating for evidence-based practices, transparently disclosing potential conflicts of interest, and actively combatting misinformation. As trusted figures in the realm of health discussions, influencers have the capacity to shape narratives and encourage ethical practices that prioritize individual well-being and foster informed health choices. By recognizing and embracing this responsibility, they can contribute to a more health-conscious society that seeks wellness through a discerning, informed approach rather than through alluring—yet potentially dangerous—myths.

10.2. Balancing Freedom with Accountability

In the modern landscape of health and wellness, the challenge of balancing freedom with accountability has never been more crucial. Individuals today are presented with a plethora of health information, particularly regarding alternative remedies like apricot seeds for cancer treatment. While this surge of information empowers consumers and grants them agency over their health choices, it also places them at considerable risk for misinformation, potentially leading to harmful consequences. Therefore, cultivating a nuanced understanding of this balance is essential to ensure that individuals can navigate these choices safely and effectively.

The concept of health freedom is foundational in many democratic societies, where individuals are encouraged to explore treatment options that resonate with their beliefs and personal experiences. This freedom allows for a diverse range of health practices to flourish, from traditional medicine to alternative therapies. However, with this freedom comes the ethical obligation to ensure that individuals are not led astray by unsubstantiated claims or misguided narratives. Misinformation, particularly as it pertains to the effectiveness of natural treatments like apricot seeds, raises questions around individual agency and the responsibility to protect public health.

Navigating this dynamic requires a multifaceted approach, addressing both the individual's right to make informed choices and the collective responsibility of health communicators and institutions to provide accurate, evidence-based information. Public health officials, medical practitioners, and health advocates play vital roles in this ecosystem, fostering a climate of informed decision-making that prioritizes safety. Awareness campaigns can help educate the public about the potential risks associated with unregulated alternative treatments, amplifying the importance of critical thinking and evidence-based health choices.

As consumers increasingly turn to the internet and social media for health advice, the potential for anecdotal evidence to overshadow established scientific findings becomes prominent. The virality of personal testimonials regarding the purported benefits of apricot seeds can create an environment where emotional narratives govern decision-making, often at the expense of rational inquiry. In this context, health advocates and professionals must commit to communicating transparently about the available evidence, ensuring that patients understand both the potential benefits and the inherent risks associated with any treatment they consider.

Furthermore, it is vital to address the role of personal autonomy in the context of accountability. While individuals should have the freedom to pursue alternative treatments, they must also be educated about the implications of their choices—especially when those choices involve unregulated products like apricot seeds. Encouraging informed consent reinforces the notion that health decisions should be made collaboratively between patients and healthcare providers, fostering a partnership built on trust and shared responsibility.

Creating a framework that emphasizes both freedom and accountability also calls for the involvement of policymakers. Legislative measures can help safeguard individuals from misleading claims while allowing space for alternative practices within regulated frameworks. Regulations around marketing, education, and consumer protection create an environment where individuals can explore diverse health paths without being exposed to harmful misinformation.

Ultimately, achieving a balance between freedom and accountability necessitates collaboration among various stakeholders in the healthcare ecosystem. Educators, practitioners, public health officials, and consumers must engage in dialogues that prioritize informed decision-making, transparency, and the collective pursuit of safety and well-being. Through this collaborative approach, we can ensure that health choices reflect both personal autonomy and the responsible dissemination of accurate information.

In conclusion, the imperative to balance freedom with accountability in health choices underscores a commitment to safeguarding public health while honoring individual autonomy. As we continue to navigate the evolving landscape of health information, let us strive for a community that embraces informed decision-making grounded in evidence—ultimately empowering individuals to make wise health choices for lifelong wellness.

10.3. What Do Practitioners Owe Their Patients?

To the patients, practitioners owe a constellation of ethical responsibilities that transcend the mere provision of medical services. This is particularly pronounced in the realm of alternative treatments, such as the controversial narrative surrounding apricot seeds as a remedy for cancer. In the delicate interplay of hope, trust, and health outcomes, practitioners must establish a foundation of integrity that prioritizes the well-being of their patients while fostering informed decision-making.

At the heart of practitioners' obligations is the principle of informed consent. Patients must understand the potential benefits and risks associated with any treatment plan, whether conventional or alternative. This responsibility necessitates clear communication, as practitioners must present information in a manner that is accessible and comprehensible, allowing individuals to weigh their options critically. When engaging with unverified remedies like apricot seeds, practitioners should ensure that patients are aware of the lack of scientific support for such treatments and the accompanying risks, including the real danger of cyanide poisoning. This transparency cultivates trust and reinforces the ethical imperative to safeguard patients' health.

Moreover, practitioners must recognize their role as educators in the health landscape. It is not enough to provide treatment; they must also empower patients with knowledge. This involves demystifying the processes surrounding health interventions, educating patients on how to evaluate health claims, and encouraging them to seek information from reputable sources. By fostering health literacy, practitioners equip their patients to navigate the complexities of health information, especially in an era characterized by the rampant spread of misinformation. In light of the appeal of natural remedies, practitioners should endeavor to guide their patients in making choices that are both safe and evidence-based.

Another essential obligation is the ethical commitment to avoid conflicts of interest when discussing alternative treatments. Practitioners must be vigilant in disclosing any affiliations or financial ties to the products they may recommend. This integrity ensures that patients receive unbiased information, free from the influence of commercial interests that could steer them toward unproven and potentially harmful therapies. For example, when addressing the allure of apricot seeds, practitioners should prioritize evidence-based recommendations, delineating clearly why certain products might not be advisable despite their marketing as natural health solutions.

Additionally, practitioners are responsible for advocating for their patients. This advocacy extends beyond the clinical setting, encouraging patients to seek second opinions and explore various treatment options. In instilling a sense of agency in their patients, practitioners empower individuals to be active participants in their health care decisions. This collaborative dynamic can foster greater satisfaction and confidence among patients, particularly those facing serious illnesses who may grapple with feelings of helplessness.

As healthcare professionals navigate the ethical landscape, they must also engage in reflective practices that consider the broader implications of their actions. Attending to social determinants of health— such as socioeconomic status, cultural beliefs, and access to resources —can enhance their understanding of patient experiences and the environment from which they seek help. This awareness can foster empathy and inform the recommendations made, tailoring advice to fit the individual context of each patient.

Moreover, the ethics of practice demand that practitioners remain open to dialogue about alternative treatments, recognizing that patients may gravitate toward options that resonate with their beliefs or cultural practices. While it is fundamental to advocate for conventional approaches based on scientific evidence, practitioners should remain respectful of patients' inquiries into alternative solutions. Engaging in these discussions can create room for education and informed decision-making while maintaining the trust between practitioner and patient.

In conclusion, practitioners owe their patients a profound ethical commitment that encompasses informed consent, education, advocacy, and unwavering integrity. The landscape of health information can be treacherous, particularly concerning alternative remedies like apricot seeds. Therefore, fostering an environment of transparency and empowerment is pivotal in ensuring that patients navigate their health journeys through a lens of informed choice. By prioritizing these ideals, practitioners can build healthier relationships with their patients, guiding them toward wise health choices rooted in integrity, evidence, and personal agency. Ultimately, the ethical responsibilities of practitioners must align with the goal of promoting lifelong wellness, grounded in informed, evidence-based decisions that prioritize patient safety and empowerment.

10.4. Ethics in Health Journalism

The emergence of ethics in health journalism has become increasingly vital in the context of a fast-paced information era marked by the rise of alternative treatments, like apricot seeds as claimed cancer cures. Health journalism serves as a bridge between scientific research, medical practice, and public awareness, playing an indispensable role in shaping how health information is communicated to the wider public. The ethical implications of health reporting cannot be overstated, especially when it comes to the accuracy, reliability, and consequences of disseminating health-related claims.

A fundamental ethical consideration in health journalism is the duty to provide accurate and evidence-based information. Journalists must ensure that the claims they present are grounded in scientific research and supported by credible sources. In the case of apricot seeds, numerous claims about their supposed cancer-fighting properties circulate in various media formats. However, without rigorous investigation and validation, these claims can mislead individuals seeking legitimate health solutions. The potential harm that can result from promoting unverified remedies highlights the critical importance of journalism that adheres to evidence-based standards.

Moreover, health journalists bear the responsibility of contextualizing information by examining the broader implications of health claims. They must delve into the scientific consensus surrounding treatments and address the associated risks of alternative options. For apricot seeds, the inherent risks of cyanide toxicity resulting from amygdalin consumption should be prominently featured alongside any reported benefits. This comprehensive approach empowers readers to weigh the pros and cons and make informed health choices.

Sensationalism in health journalism poses an additional ethical challenge. The quest for increased readership often leads to exaggeration, oversimplification, or sensational presentation of scientific findings. Headlines that tout "miracle cures" or "breakthrough treatments" can misrepresent complex health issues, ultimately compromising the integrity of the information conveyed. Journalists must uphold a commitment to responsible reporting by avoiding inflammatory language and focusing on clear, factual communication that reflects the intricacies of health topics.

Furthermore, ethical health journalism necessitates transparency regarding conflicts of interest. Health journalists must disclose any affiliations or partnerships that may influence the stories they produce, promoting trust and credibility within the audience. This is especially pertinent when addressing topics related to alternative treatments, such as apricot seeds, where the interests of advocates can intersect with journalists' narratives. Consumers have the right to be aware of any potential biases that may affect the information they are receiving.

Additionally, health journalists must engage in critical self-reflection to recognize their own biases and the caveats surrounding the narratives they construct. The dynamic between public perception and scientific evidence can be complex. Journalists should strive to present a balanced view of alternative treatments, acknowledging the emotional narratives that often accompany personal testimonials while reinforcing the need to rely on proven, evidence-based approaches to health.

Public engagement with health information is another significant ethical consideration for health journalism. Journalists have an obligation to facilitate inclusive conversations that consider the perspectives of diverse communities. Different cultures may harbor distinct beliefs regarding health and wellness, particularly when discussing natural remedies. By incorporating various viewpoints and emphasizing cultural sensitivity, health journalists can bridge gaps and foster understanding around health narratives that resonate with different audiences.

Lastly, health journalism must advocate for accountability among both health influencers and practitioners who promote alternative treatments. Drawing attention to instances where unverified claims can lead to adverse health outcomes—such as those associated with apricot seeds—helps ensure that ethical standards are upheld across the healthcare landscape. By fostering transparency and accountability, health journalists can appropriately challenge narratives that may inadvertently cause harm to individuals and communities.

In summary, the ethical dimensions of health journalism bear profound significance in a world where misinformation can drastically affect public health decisions. Journalists are tasked with the responsibility to uphold accuracy, transparency, and integrity in conveying health-related information, particularly concerning controversial topics like apricot seeds. By remaining committed to evidence-based reporting that considers the broader implications of health claims, journalists can cultivate an informed public capable of making wise, safe health choices. As the landscape of health continues to evolve, the ethics of health journalism will play a pivotal role in nurturing a society that prioritizes patient safety, well-being, and informed decision-making.

10.5. Learning from Past Mistakes

In the ever-evolving landscape of health information, the importance of learning from past mistakes cannot be overstated. Historical examples of healthcare missteps serve as poignant reminders of the potential consequences of unchecked misinformation, especially when it pertains to alternative treatments that draw considerable public interest, like apricot seeds as a supposed solution for cancer. Understanding these past failures sheds light on how to navigate the challenges that arise within health communication and the complexities of treatment decisions.

One of the most notable examples of health misinformation impacting public health is the promotion of laetrile, derived from apricot seeds and marketed as vitamin B17. In the mid-20th century, this compound gained notoriety as a supposed cure for cancer, despite a lack of scientific evidence to support its efficacy. Patients, often desperate for hope amidst devastating diagnoses, turned to laetrile in droves, influenced by poignant testimonials and the allure of natural remedies. The consequences of this public belief were dire. Many individuals who relied on laetrile as a treatment for cancer experienced adverse health effects, including severe cyanide poisoning. This tragic misunderstanding highlights the dangers that can arise when narratives overstate the benefits of alternative treatments without backing from rigorous scientific validation.

The rise of the anti-vaccine movement further emphasizes the critical need to learn from past mistakes in health communication. The debunked link between the MMR vaccine and autism, based on a fraudulent study published in the late 1990s, led to widespread vaccine hesitancy and resulted in preventable outbreaks of diseases. This incident underscores how misinformation can gain traction, propelled by emotional narratives and fear, ultimately jeopardizing public health outcomes. Learning from this mistake stresses the importance of transparency in scientific research, as well as the need for healthcare professionals to engage with the public in truthful, empathetic conversations that address concerns robustly and clearly.

In examining the impacts of these past missteps, it becomes evident that the healthcare community must prioritize proactive strategies to combat misinformation. This involves educating the public about the necessity of evidence-based medicine and the potential dangers associated with unregulated alternative treatments. Effective communication should not only share scientific insights but also dismantle myths surrounding popular trends, providing context for why certain remedies, despite their allure, lack empirical support.

Moreover, fostering a culture of critical thinking is essential for empowering individuals to discern fact from fiction in health claims. Past failures often resulted from an overreliance on anecdotal evidence without sufficient scrutiny of the available scientific literature. Advancing health literacy initiatives—educating individuals on how to evaluate health information critically and navigate the digital landscape effectively—can significantly mitigate the risks posed by misinformation.

Engaging diverse communities in health discussions is equally important. Acknowledging the histories, beliefs, and values held by various populations helps tailor communications that resonate meaningfully, fostering trust. As we reflect on past mistakes, we ought to embrace the principle of inclusivity, ensuring that all voices are heard and respected, particularly in discussions surrounding alternative treatments.

Additionally, stakeholders—ranging from healthcare providers to policymakers—must work collaboratively to promote accuracy in health communication. Advocates for public health must influence policy changes that prioritize evidence-based practices and regulate the claims made by alternative treatments. By demanding accountability from both individuals and organizations who propagate misleading health information, the risks of misinformation can be significantly reduced.

This call for learning from past mistakes extends beyond mere reflection; it demands action. Harnessing the lessons derived from previous missteps around alternative treatments like apricot seeds guides the cultivation of a more informed and vigilant public, capable of navigating the complexities of health choices.

In conclusion, the imperative to learn from past mistakes shapes our collective understanding of health communication and informs future decisions regarding alternative treatments. The cases of apricot seeds and laetrile provide crucial insights into the potential consequences of sweeping claims devoid of scientific support. By prioritizing education, fostering critical thinking, and advocating for transparency, we can build a healthcare environment where informed choices prevail —a vital endeavor in the ever-changing landscape of health and wellness. Learning from past mistakes not only shapes our present but also determines our path toward a healthier, more informed future.

11. The Psychological Draw of Natural Cures

11.1. Understanding the Appeal of Nature

Understanding the appeal of nature serves as a cornerstone in the exploration of health narratives, specifically regarding alternative treatments and their emotional resonance with individuals. The notion that nature holds intrinsic healing properties is deeply rooted in cultural beliefs, historical practices, and the human desire for simplicity in navigating complex health challenges. This subchapter aims to elucidate the psychological mechanisms behind the allure of natural remedies, while also examining the implications of harnessing such sentiments in health discussions.

Human beings have long sought solace in the natural world as a source of healing and wellness. Throughout history, many cultures have relied on herbal medicine, traditional healing practices, and natural ingredients to address health issues. This connection to nature epitomizes a fundamental aspect of what it means to be human: an inherent desire to harmonize with the environment and a faith that the very fabrics of nature can provide respite, relief, and recovery from ailments. This belief system illustrates why alternatives to conventional medicine—such as apricot seeds touted as cancer cures—can captivate individuals desperate for hope amidst serious health battles.

The appeal of nature is often intertwined with a yearning for self-determination in health choices. Individuals facing daunting diseases may feel a loss of control over their circumstances due to the often stark realities associated with conventional treatment approaches. In this context, the adoption of natural remedies allows patients to reclaim agency, offering them a sense of empowerment in navigating their health journeys. The narrative that a simple, humble item like an apricot seed could possess the power to heal provides a powerful emotional connection, empowering individuals to take charge of their health decisions.

Moreover, the comfort offered by the idea of natural cures provides psychological reassurance to many. In a world often marked by complexity, frustration, and uncertainty surrounding conventional medical treatments, the notion of a straightforward solution—a single entity derived from nature—can feel profoundly appealing. This psychological comfort resonates within the individual's frame of reference, allowing them to believe that healing doesn't have to be complicated; the remedy may lie just a seed away. Such simplicity is compelling, particularly when faced with the convoluted narratives of medical interventions that may not yield immediate or guaranteed results.

However, the innate longing for situations that allow easy choices can lead to uncritical acceptance of health claims surrounding natural remedies. Individuals eager for solutions may willingly bypass rigorous empirical evidence to embrace these narratives, especially when stories of miraculous recoveries circulate in public discourse. The rampant promotion of apricot seeds as alternative treatments epitomizes this phenomenon, wherein anecdotal testimonials can take precedence over scientific consensus. Moreover, confirmation bias often shapes how individuals engage with health information, swaying them toward narratives that resonate with their beliefs while disregarding contradictory evidence.

Challenging established narratives becomes a responsibility in the pursuit of educated health choices. Emphasizing the need for a balanced perspective amidst the allure of nature means reminding individuals that healing encompasses more than merely consuming a natural product. It requires understanding the complexities of health and illness, acknowledging societal influences, and making responsible decisions shaped by information and evidence rather than solely by emotional narratives.

As we strive for a balanced outlook on health choices, the dialogue must foster an understanding of both the benefits and limitations of natural remedies. While nature certainly holds valuable healing properties, individuals must also be encouraged to approach health with informed skepticism, carefully weighing options in light of scientific evidence and the realities of their health conditions. Here, the role of healthcare professionals becomes indispensable—by providing guidance on the efficacy and safety of various treatments, practitioners can create a supportive framework for individuals seeking natural alternatives, effectively translating the allure of nature into responsible health choices.

In conclusion, understanding the appeal of nature is integral to grasping why individuals gravitate toward alternative remedies, as it intersects with themes of self-determination, psychological comfort, and the emotional weight of personal narratives. While the fascination with natural cures offers a sense of empowerment, it remains crucial to root health choices in scientific understanding and proactive decision-making. By promoting thoughtful inquiry, balanced discussions, and the appreciation of nature within a broader context of health, we can cultivate a healthier discourse that respects both the wisdom of the past and the advancements of modern science.

11.2. The Quest for Self-determination in Health Choices

The quest for self-determination in health choices represents both a deeply human impulse and a significant challenge in navigating the complexities of modern healthcare. In an age where information is abundant, yet often misleading, individuals are increasingly empowered to make their own health decisions, including exploring alternatives to conventional medicine. This quest becomes particularly pronounced with the rise of narratives surrounding natural remedies like apricot seeds, which are promoted by some as a potential solution to cancer. However, the interplay of hope, misinformation, and the desire for agency can lead to unintended consequences, necessitating a closer examination of how individuals can exercise informed self-determination.

At its core, self-determination in health choices is rooted in the principles of autonomy and empowerment. Individuals naturally seek to take charge of their health and make decisions that resonate with their values and beliefs. This desire is often intensified when faced with a serious illness, as patients grapple with overwhelming medical information and treatment options. The notion that a simple, natural remedy may offer a respite from the complexities of modern medicine can be incredibly appealing. For many, the allure of apricot seeds as a cancer remedy symbolizes hope, control, and a direct connection to nature's healing properties.

However, the pursuit of this self-determination must be tempered with a commitment to informed decision-making. Individuals need to recognize the potential risks associated with alternative treatments, particularly those lacking empirical support. The case of apricot seeds serves as a cautionary tale, emphasizing the importance of discerning credible information from unverified claims. The narrative propagated by anecdotal success stories can overshadow the urgent warning issued by the scientific community regarding the dangers of cyanide poisoning. As such, individuals must actively seek out reliable resources and engage with healthcare professionals who can provide evidence-based insights, fostering a more nuanced under-standing of their options.

Psychological comfort plays a pivotal role in individuals' journeys toward self-determination. Many people are drawn to alternative treatments as a means of reclaiming agency over their health amid feelings of helplessness. This sense of control can alleviate anxieties tied to dire diagnoses, offering reassurance and a path forward. How-ever, this psychological comfort can cloud judgment, leading some to embrace remedies like apricot seeds without fully grappling with the associated risks. It is essential to strike a balance between the desire for empowerment and the necessity of grounding health decisions in factual, evidence-based information.

Challenging established narratives surrounding alternative treat-ments is also a critical component of the quest for self-determination. Individuals must learn to question the validity of sensational claims that promise simple solutions to complex health issues. The cultural tendency to trust "natural" options over conventional medicines may contribute to a pattern of uncritical acceptance in the face of compelling anecdotes. Promoting open dialogue about the limitations and realities of alternative treatments encourages critical reflection and improves decision-making, ultimately enhancing patient safety and well-being.

Moving toward a balanced perspective involves embracing the complexities inherent in health choices. Individuals should recognize that self-determination does not equate to the rejection of conventional medicine; rather, it should involve an integrated approach in which patients work collaboratively with healthcare professionals to explore all viable options. This comprehensive approach allows for a more informed decision-making process that respects personal beliefs while ensuring safety and efficacy in treatment choices.

In conclusion, the quest for self-determination in health choices signifies a fundamental aspect of human experience—our desire for agency in the face of illness. However, this quest must be approached thoughtfully, emphasizing informed decision-making, psychological comfort, critical evaluation of narratives, and a balanced perspective that integrates various treatment modalities. By empowering individuals to navigate their health journeys with knowledge and intentionality, we can foster a culture that values both autonomy and responsibility, enabling people to make wise health choices that enhance their overall well-being.

11.3. Psychological Comfort in Control Over Treatment

Psychological comfort in control over treatment serves as a foundational theme in the conversation surrounding health autonomy and decision-making, particularly in the context of alternative treatments like apricot seeds purported to combat cancer. The desire for agency in navigating one's health choices is deeply ingrained in human nature. Individuals facing serious health challenges often report feeling overwhelmed by the complexity of medical information and recommendations, leading them to seek out solutions that empower them to take charge of their care. This quest for control becomes particularly pronounced in discussions of alternative remedies, where patients yearn for a sense of agency amid the uncertainty surrounding progressive illnesses.

The psychological comfort derived from controlling health decisions stems from a human instinct to reclaim power in situations often filled with fear and vulnerability. Facing a cancer diagnosis can evoke feelings of helplessness and anxiety, prompting individuals to explore alternative solutions that offer the promise of recovery without the harsh realities often associated with conventional medicine. For many, the narrative that a simple, natural substance can facilitate healing resonates profoundly with their emotional needs. Apricot seeds, for example, might symbolize not only a potential remedy but also a broader desire to find hope amidst despair.

The sense of empowerment can manifest in various ways, such as the act of researching and selecting treatment options that align with personal beliefs. This self-determination can foster psychological resilience, as individuals feel more engaged with their health journeys. However, when the quest for control leads individuals to alternative treatments unproven by rigorous scientific evidence, the psychological comfort can turn into a double-edged sword. The appeal of apricot seeds as a cancer treatment exemplifies this dichotomy; while the seeds may symbolize empowerment and hope, reliance on such unverified remedies can also expose individuals to significant health risks, including the threat of cyanide poisoning due to amygdalin.

Moreover, health professionals must navigate the emotional landscape of patients when discussing treatment options. Acknowledging the human desire for self-determination is essential when guiding individuals toward evidence-based practices. This requires practitioners to engage in compassionate communication that validates patients' fears and aspirations while also providing accurate, scientifically supported information. When addressing the appeal of apricot seeds, healthcare providers must underscore not only the risks associated with their consumption but also the secure, effective alternatives available through conventional medical treatment—a move that emphasizes both safety and support.

The role of psychological comfort in self-determination also resonates within broader societal narratives surrounding health and well-being. The cultural values attributed to natural remedies often give rise to a tension between the allure of nature and the realities of rigorous medical practice. In many communities, the belief in the healing properties of natural substances drives the market for alternative treatments, creating a space where anecdotal evidence triumphs over scientific rigor. This disparity reflects a broader struggle to balance traditional beliefs with contemporary medical understanding.

Ultimately, psychological comfort in control over treatment poses a complex challenge within the landscape of health decision-making. It invites a deeper exploration of how the interplay of hope, fear, and agency influences the choices individuals make in the face of serious illnesses. While fostering self-determination and autonomy is vital to improving patient engagement and outcomes, it is equally important to ground these desires in critical thinking and scientific evidence. For individuals interested in alternative treatments, striking a balance between hope and caution becomes paramount.

In conclusion, the quest for psychological comfort in controlling health decisions embodies a nuanced facet of patient advocacy. While the search for empowerment is a fundamental aspect of the human experience, it must be paired with responsible decision-making rooted in scientific understanding. The conversation surrounding apricot seeds—and alternative treatments in general—highlights the importance of fostering informed autonomy that prioritizes safety and efficacy in navigating the complex health landscape. By embracing a balanced perspective, individuals can optimize their health decisions while remaining vigilant against the siren call of unverified remedies.

11.4. Challenging Established Narratives

Challenging established narratives serves as a crucial aspect of fostering informed health decisions, particularly in the realm of alternative treatments like apricot seeds for cancer. The narratives surrounding natural remedies often emerge from a complex interplay of historical beliefs, emotional appeals, cultural heritage, and the desire for simple solutions to complex health problems. While these narratives can provide comfort and hope, they may also propagate misinformation and distract from evidence-based approaches that prioritize safety and efficacy. Therefore, to navigate health choices responsibly, it becomes imperative to scrutinize and challenge established narratives, particularly those that lack scientific validation.

The rise of alternative treatments is often rooted in a historical context that revered natural remedies. Ancient healing practices, which relied on herbs and plants for their medicinal properties, have been passed down through generations, fostering a deep-seated belief in nature's power to heal. However, contemporary claims, such as those that apricot seeds can cure cancer, frequently oversimplify the complexities of medical science. The danger lies in allowing narratives fueled by anecdotal evidence or individual testimonials to supersede rigorous scientific inquiry, an inclination that can lead to misguided health decisions.

One essential step in challenging established narratives is to promote critical engagement with health information. Individuals must be encouraged to question the validity of health claims and seek out reliable sources of information. This involves examining whether there is scientific consensus regarding the efficacy of a treatment and whether claims are substantiated by empirical research. For instance, while personal testimonials about the benefits of apricot seeds may proliferate online, these must be assessed against the considerable body of scientific literature that categorically dismisses their effectiveness and highlights the associated risks of cyanide exposure.

Cultivating a health-literate society involves instilling the ability to discern credible sources from questionable ones. Public health education campaigns can enhance this literacy by providing guidance on how to evaluate health claims critically. Engaging individuals through workshops, accessible online resources, and community programs can foster the skills necessary to navigate health information wisely. Ultimately, the goal is to empower individuals to make informed choices grounded in facts rather than feelings, ensuring that narratives surrounding health treatments are scrutinized rigorously.

Furthermore, challenging established narratives requires a concerted effort among healthcare professionals, researchers, educators, and advocates. This joint endeavor can amplify the importance of evidence-based medicine while addressing the allure of natural remedies. By actively participating in dialogues surrounding alternative treatments, health professionals can provide scientifically validated perspectives that counteract misleading claims. Additionally, offering patients insight into the historical context behind these narratives can foster a wider understanding, emphasizing how cultural beliefs can shape perceptions of health.

The role of social media cannot be overlooked in the discussion of established narratives. The digital landscape provides a platform for both the dissemination of credible health information and the rapid spread of misinformation. Leveraging social media to promote narratives grounded in science becomes imperative for healthcare organizations and advocates. During health crises, such as the rise of interest in apricot seeds, ensuring that accurate information is amplified while countering false narratives is essential in guiding public understanding.

In addition, regulatory agencies must reflect on their communication strategies to address alternative treatments effectively. By providing clear guidelines and issuing warnings about the unsubstantiated claims surrounding certain remedies, these agencies can help reestablish a more reliable narrative about health choices. When consumers understand that specific alternative treatments are not backed by scientific evidence, they are less likely to gravitate toward these options, ultimately fostering a safer healthcare landscape.

In conclusion, challenging established narratives is a vital component of fostering informed health decisions, particularly concerning alternative treatments like apricot seeds. This endeavor necessitates a commitment to critical engagement, education, and collaboration among health professionals, educators, and community advocates. As we work to navigate the complexities of health information, let us prioritize science over sensationalism, ensuring that our understanding of health choices is guided by evidence, integrity, and safety. By embracing this approach, we support the pursuit of well-being and empower individuals to make responsible health decisions that prioritize their safety and wellness.

11.5. Towards a Balanced Perspective

As we delve into the importance of a balanced perspective in the discourse surrounding health, specifically regarding the myths surrounding apricot seeds as cancer treatments, we are reminded that the conversation must evolve beyond simplistic narratives or emotional appeals. It has become increasingly clear that navigating this topic requires a nuanced understanding of the interplay between scientific research, historical practices, and the psychological factors that drive individuals towards particular health beliefs.

At the core of our inquiry lies the recognition that while alternative remedies often appeal to deeply ingrained historical traditions and personal narratives of healing, they must be scrutinized through a lens of critical inquiry grounded in scientific validation. Embracing a balanced perspective allows us to honor the cultural and historical context of natural remedies without losing sight of the necessity for rigorous research and empirical evidence to support health claims.

For example, the narrative surrounding apricot seeds hinges on centuries of lore that romanticizes natural treatments. Many individuals are drawn to the idea that a simple seed, derived from nature, could provide a cure for a disease as formidable as cancer. This sentiment taps into the psychological desire for control and empowerment in health decisions, allowing patients to feel proactive in their care. Yet, it is vital to counter this with robust discussions about the scientific consensus that unequivocally states the risks associated with consuming these seeds, namely the potential for cyanide poisoning.

In fostering a balanced perspective, we must acknowledge the psychological comfort people derive from narratives of natural healing. However, this should not come at the expense of informed decision-making. It is the responsibility of healthcare providers, public health officials, and advocates to communicate the complexities of these narratives thoughtfully, promoting a culture that values safety and efficacy over hope-driven myths. Engaging with patients about the limitations and risks of alternative treatments empowers them to make choices that are rooted in evidence and personal safety rather than anecdotal success stories.

Moreover, it is essential to emphasize the importance of education in health literacy. By equipping individuals with the tools to critically evaluate health information, we can create a more informed public discourse surrounding health practices. Patients should be encouraged to ask questions, seek out reliable sources, and approach health decisions with a discerning eye. This empowerment not only enhances individuals' capacity to navigate their health journeys but also aids in dispelling myths stemming from misinformation.

Importantly, open scientific discourse plays a crucial role in our quest towards a balanced perspective. Encouraging both experts and laypeople to engage in discussions about alternative treatments fosters an environment of inquiry and exchange, allowing for the ebb and flow of ideas grounded in both personal experience and empirical research. Scientific dialogue should be accessible, inviting individuals from diverse backgrounds to contribute to ongoing conversations about health while reinforcing the importance of robust evidence in guiding choices.

As we bridge the gaps between experts and the public, we highlight the necessity of collaboration across disciplines to foster a comprehensive understanding of health. Health communicators, researchers, practitioners, and advocates must work together to share resources, knowledge, and experiences in a manner that is inclusive and respectful of individual beliefs while simultaneously prioritizing safety and scientific credibility.

Ultimately, striving for a balanced perspective involves recognizing the intricate web of interests, beliefs, and values that shape health narratives. This pursuit requires humility and a commitment to continuous learning as we navigate the complexities inherent in health decisions. By fostering an environment that encourages critical inquiry, embraces shared experiences, and empowers individuals, we work towards creating a health dialogue that champions informed choices and the quest for wellness without falling prey to the perils of misinformation.

In conclusion, embracing a balanced perspective in our discussions about apricot seeds and alternative remedies involves a multifaceted approach that emphasizes evidence, education, and respectful dialogue. By grounding our conversations in solid scientific inquiry while acknowledging the emotional and cultural factors that inform health choices, we can create a healthier dialogue about wellness— a dialogue that champions informed choices, prioritizes safety, and ultimately fosters a more resilient society in the face of health challenges.

12. Distilling Truth in a Sea of Information

12.1. The Challenge of Information Saturation

The challenge of information saturation in today's world is becoming increasingly evident, particularly regarding health-related topics. With a deluge of data available on the internet, individuals are bombarded with conflicting information about treatments, remedies, and health trends. This phenomenon poses significant risks, especially in the context of alternative therapies such as apricot seeds claimed to have potential cancer-fighting properties. The allure of these simple, natural solutions may captivate those seeking hope, but without careful navigation, the consequences of misinformation can be dire.

Understanding information saturation begins with recognizing the sheer volume of available content. Social media, online forums, health blogs, and news outlets contribute to a 24/7 cycle of information flow. While this accessibility can facilitate knowledge-sharing, it can also lead to confusion, as contradictory messages vie for attention. For instance, an individual may come across compelling testimonials extolling the virtues of apricot seeds alongside robust scientific critiques of their efficacy and safety. The saturation of differing claims complicates decision-making processes, as people may struggle to determine which sources are credible amid an overwhelming sea of information.

One notable consequence of this saturation is the prevalence of misinformation. The rapid spread of unverified health claims is exacerbated by social media algorithms prioritizing sensationalized content, leading to the viral propagation of certain narratives. In the case of apricot seeds, the narrative that they can cure cancer has gained significant traction among certain populations, fueled by anecdotal evidence and emotional stories. This powerful appeal can lead individuals to overlook or dismiss the scientific consensus that categorically rejects such claims, resulting in a disconnect between perceived and actual realities. The resulting misinformation can drive individuals toward choices that may ultimately compromise their health.

Furthermore, information saturation can foster cognitive biases, such as confirmation bias, wherein individuals selectively attend to information corroborating their preexisting beliefs. This tendency exacerbates the challenge of discerning truth from fiction, as individuals may gravitate toward narratives that align with their desires—such as the hope that apricot seeds can provide a simple, natural solution to a complex disease. In seeking out favorable evidence, they may inadvertently reinforce their misconceptions, perpetuating cycles of misinformation.

Addressing the challenge of information saturation requires a multifaceted approach. First, fostering critical thinking skills among individuals becomes paramount. Education initiatives focused on developing health literacy empower consumers to assess the credibility of sources, critically evaluate claims, and recognize potential red flags in health messaging. Individuals must be equipped with the knowledge needed to differentiate between anecdotal testimonials and rigorous scientific research, allowing them to navigate the complex landscape of health information more confidently.

Moreover, healthcare professionals and policymakers play a crucial role in combating misinformation and promoting responsible health messaging. By actively engaging in public discussions, providing accurate information, and collaborating with trusted influencers, they can guide individuals toward evidence-based practices and dispel harmful myths. This proactive approach is essential in cultivating an environment where individuals feel safe seeking guidance from reputable sources rather than relying on unverified claims.

Additionally, leveraging technology to track health-related information and promote transparency can aid in addressing information saturation. Initiatives such as apps that provide access to credible scientific research, health databases, and expert reference materials can equip individuals with the tools necessary to verify claims they encounter online. By centralizing reliable resources, consumers can make informed decisions while navigating the sea of information that constantly bombards them.

In conclusion, the challenge of information saturation presents significant hurdles in the quest for informed health choices. As the lure of simple solutions such as apricot seeds can captivate a yearning public, the risks of misinformation cannot be ignored. Promoting critical thinking, empowering individuals through education, and leveraging technology can foster an environment where truth prevails in health discourse. As society navigates this complex landscape, a concerted effort to prioritize evidence-based information while addressing the emotional narratives surrounding health treatments will be essential in fostering wise health choices for lifelong wellness.

12.2. Building Critical Thinking Skills

The ability to build critical thinking skills is essential in navigating the complex landscape of health information, especially in light of the rampant misinformation surrounding alternative treatments like apricot seeds touted as cancer cures. In an age where individuals often turn to the internet for answers to their health questions, enhancing one's capacity for critical thought emerges as a fundamental tool for discerning fact from fiction.

At the heart of critical thinking lies the ability to analyze and evaluate information rigorously. This involves questioning the credibility of the sources from which information is derived. Are these sources reputable? Do they present information grounded in empirical research, or are they based on anecdotal evidence and personal testimonials? By fostering a habit of inquiry, individuals can develop a more discerning approach to health claims, which is particularly salient when confronted with the stories and emotional appeals often found in discussions about alternative remedies. For instance, in the case of apricot seeds, claims of miraculous healing must be scrutinized against the backdrop of scientific research that highlights their potential risks, including cyanide toxicity.

Another essential aspect of building critical thinking skills is engaging with diverse perspectives. Health narratives are often shaped by cultural beliefs and emotional needs, which can cloud judgment. Encouraging individuals to seek diverse viewpoints can help unveil biases and open up discussions that consider multiple angles. When individuals are exposed to a range of opinions—from traditional medical practices to alternative treatments—they become better equipped to navigate the intricate web of health information and make informed decisions.

Moreover, individuals should be encouraged to engage in reflective practices when evaluating health claims. This reflective process involves taking a step back and considering the motivations behind particular narratives. Are the claims driven by genuine concern for patient well-being, or are they motivated by commercial interests? Understanding the context in which health information is presented can help individuals distinguish between valuable insights and self-serving claims, especially in cases where products like apricot seeds are marketed without adequate disclaimers about their health risks.

Education plays an undeniable role in fostering critical thinking skills. Integrative health literacy programs that emphasize the importance of evaluating information critically can equip individuals with the tools needed to navigate the deluge of health-related content. These programs should focus on teaching individuals how to assess reliability, recognize potential biases, and evaluate evidence. By instilling these skills at an early age or through ongoing adult education initiatives, communities can promote informed citizenry capable of challenging misinformation and making sound health choices.

As advancements in technology continue to shape how individuals access health information, it is vital to leverage these tools effectively. Online resources and digital platforms can facilitate the dissemination of accurate health information while promoting critical engagement. Health organizations and advocacy groups should be proactive in providing clear and accessible data on various health topics, including evidence-based information about alternative treatments and their risks. By harnessing the power of digital platforms, they can reach wider audiences, particularly populations that may be more susceptible to misinformation.

Additionally, encouraging open scientific discourse plays a significant role in fostering critical thinking. Creating inclusive environments where healthcare professionals can communicate with the public about health issues, including the risks associated with alternative treatments like apricot seeds, allows for the exchange of ideas and promotes understanding. Such discourse can help demystify complex topics and clarify misconceptions that may arise from sensationalized narratives.

The role of experts in health communication cannot be overlooked; bridging gaps between scientists, practitioners, and the public enhances the exchange of valuable information and encourages accountability. By connecting individuals with credible experts who can contextualize health claims and provide evidence-based guidance, the community can forge a stronger foundation of trust—one that seeks to enhance informed decision-making and critical evaluation of health narratives.

Ultimately, the capacity to build critical thinking skills is a vital cornerstone in navigating the complex web of health information. By fostering inquiry, engaging with diverse perspectives, and emphasizing education, individuals can emerge equipped to challenge misinformation, make informed health choices, and advocate for their well-being. In the face of claims surrounding hazardous alternative treatments, like those involving apricot seeds, empowering individuals with the tools necessary for critical evaluation enhances public health outcomes and fosters a community committed to safe and effective health practices.

12.3. Role of Education in Health Literacy

Education plays a pivotal role in enhancing health literacy, particularly in the context of understanding and evaluating alternative treatments like apricot seeds for cancer. As the proliferation of health information continues rapidly in the digital age, the ability to discern credible information from misinformation becomes increasingly essential. By fostering comprehensive education and critical thinking, we can empower individuals to make informed health choices that prioritize safety and efficacy.

Health literacy encompasses not only the ability to read and comprehend health-related materials but also the capacity to critically engage with this information. It includes understanding medical terminology, treatment options, and the implications of various approaches. Empowering individuals with health literacy strengthens their ability to evaluate claims about alternative treatments, allowing them to discern between scientifically validated therapies and those lacking empirical support. For instance, individuals equipped with health literacy skills can analyze the risks associated with consuming apricot seeds and the potential adverse effects of cyanide toxicity stemming from amygdalin.

In educational settings, it is crucial to incorporate topics that specifically address alternative medicine and the potential pitfalls associated with unverified treatments. Curricula that emphasize critical thinking and discernment in health information can help students, patients, and community members navigate the complexities of health choices. This education should be accessible and culturally sensitive, recognizing diverse backgrounds and beliefs surrounding health practices. Integrating real-life scenarios, case studies, and interactive discussions can make the learning process engaging and relevant.

Healthcare professionals play a key role in promoting health literacy. By fostering open communication with patients, providers can facilitate discussions that demystify health information while addressing concerns about alternative remedies. Encouraging inquiries and providing understandable explanations helps patients feel empowered to actively participate in their care. For example, when discussing the risks of apricot seeds, healthcare providers should offer clear evidence and guidance, allowing patients to make decisions based on knowledge rather than fear or misinformation.

Technology also offers innovative opportunities to enhance health literacy. Digital platforms provide various resources that individuals can access easily—such as online databases, webinars, and informative websites. These tools can be harnessed to create educational campaigns that promote critical thinking and evidence-based practices. For instance, the integration of user-friendly applications that guide individuals in evaluating health claims can empower patients to seek information that is reliable and grounded in scientific literature.

Moreover, health education should extend beyond individual patients. Community engagement initiatives allow for broader discussions around health literacy, reaching diverse audiences who may be more susceptible to misinformation regarding alternative treatments. Public health campaigns aimed at empowering communities to engage with health narratives critically can nurture a culture of informed health choices. Workshops, town halls, and community outreach programs can serve as platforms for disseminating accurate information and fostering health literacy on a larger scale.

In conclusion, the role of education in health literacy is essential for challenging the appeal of alternative treatments like apricot seeds. By fostering critical thinking, enhancing communication, utilizing technology, and engaging with communities, we can empower individuals to navigate health choices with informed confidence. Education equips patients with the skills necessary to evaluate the risks and benefits of various remedies, ultimately promoting safety and well-being in their health journeys. As we continue to explore the evolving landscape of health information, the commitment to education must remain steadfast, guiding individuals toward lifelong wellness and informed health advocacy.

12.4. Encouraging Open Scientific Discourse

Encouraging open scientific discourse in the realm of health—especially regarding alternative treatments like apricot seeds—serves as an essential strategy in promoting informed decision-making. As misinformation proliferates in the digital age, fostering an environment where evidence-based discussions can thrive becomes imperative. Open scientific discourse encourages individuals to engage critically with health narratives, allowing them to weigh the benefits and risks of various treatments against a backdrop of empirical knowledge.

One fundamental aspect of encouraging open scientific discourse is creating platforms where researchers, healthcare professionals, and the public can engage in dialogue. Community forums, workshops, and public lectures offer opportunities for sharing information, dispelling myths, and addressing concerns about alternative treatments. By fostering these open dialogues, individuals are afforded the chance to ask questions and gain insights into complex health issues, ultimately empowering them to make more informed choices.

Moreover, educational initiatives that highlight the importance of scientific reasoning can cultivate a culture of inquiry. By teaching individuals how to interpret research findings, evaluate the credibility of sources, and distinguish between evidence and anecdote, we equip them with the tools necessary to engage in health discussions meaningfully. For instance, communities can benefit from workshops that instruct participants on how to evaluate claims surrounding apricot seeds and other alternative treatments critically, emphasizing the need to consult reliable sources and medical professionals.

Engaging healthcare professionals in promoting open scientific discourse is also critical. When doctors and scientists actively participate in discussions surrounding alternative treatments, they can provide evidence-based perspectives that rebalance the conversation. Their involvement can help clarify misconceptions and highlight the importance of adhering to established medical protocols while respecting patients' rights to explore other options. Healthcare providers should strive to maintain open lines of communication with patients and recognize the emotional weight that discussions about alternative remedies carry.

Additionally, the role of digital platforms cannot be underestimated in fostering open scientific discourse. Social media, blogs, and online discussion forums can serve as vehicles for disseminating accurate health information and creating communities where individuals can share their experiences. However, these platforms also require vigilant moderation to ensure that misleading claims do not dominate the conversation. Public health organizations and advocacy groups must take the initiative to utilize digital channels effectively, promoting accurate narratives while countering the allure of sensationalized anecdotes.

Furthermore, encouraging collaboration between researchers and health communicators can strengthen the integrity of public health messaging. By working together, these stakeholders can translate complex scientific findings into accessible language that resonates with diverse audiences. This collaboration can enhance public understanding of alternative treatments and the scientific reasoning behind evidence-based practices, leading to more meaningful discussions surrounding health choices.

As we strive to create open scientific discourse, it is essential to leverage the diverse perspectives and experiences that shape health narratives. Engaging patients and community members in discussions allows health advocates to appreciate the cultural, emotional, and psychological factors that inform their beliefs and health choices. This understanding helps foster empathy while encouraging a collaborative approach where individuals feel valued and heard.

In conclusion, encouraging open scientific discourse serves as a powerful tool in combatting misinformation and promoting informed health decision-making. By creating inclusive platforms for discussion, enhancing health literacy, and fostering collaboration among stakeholders, we can build an environment that nurtures evidence-based discussions about alternative treatments like apricot seeds. Ultimately, this discourse empowers individuals, enabling them to navigate their health journeys with knowledge, confidence, and a commitment to their well-being. As we cultivate an open and inquisitive approach to health conversations, we pave the way for a future where informed choices reign supreme, leading to better health outcomes for individuals and communities alike.

12.5. Bridging Gaps Between Experts and the Public

Bridging the gaps between experts and the public is essential in today's complex landscape of health information, particularly as alternative treatments such as apricot seeds attract attention and controversy. The digital age has transformed how health information is shared and consumed, creating unique challenges and opportunities for facilitating effective communication. As misinformation proliferates across social media platforms, it is imperative to cultivate strong connections between healthcare professionals, researchers, and the general public in order to promote informed decision-making and patient safety.

One foundational element of bridging these gaps is fostering trust and transparency. Healthcare professionals must engage actively with the communities they serve, providing clear and accessible information. This engagement is essential for addressing misconceptions and ensuring that the public receives accurate health guidance, particularly when discussing alternative treatments. In the case of apricot seeds, which are often marketed as a natural remedy for cancer, experts must openly share the scientific consensus on their efficacy and the significant risks associated with their consumption, such as cyanide toxicity. Transparent communication not only builds credibility but also fosters a collaborative environment where individuals feel empowered to ask questions and seek guidance.

Moreover, creating accessible and relatable communication strategies can enhance public understanding of complex health topics. Using plain language, avoiding medical jargon, and employing visual aids can help demystify scientific information. This approach encourages dialogue and invites public participation in discussions surrounding health choices. For instance, healthcare providers can utilize community workshops, informational pamphlets, or social media campaigns to articulate the potential risks of apricot seeds clearly and provide evidence-based alternatives for cancer treatment. By presenting information that resonates with the audience's experiences and values, experts can bridge the gap and foster greater engagement.

Additionally, leveraging technology offers significant potential for effective communication. Digital platforms can serve as valuable tools for disseminating health information. Developing mobile applications or websites that provide evidence-based resources, interactive tools for assessing health claims, and forums for community discussion can empower individuals to navigate the digital health landscape effectively. Partnering with tech experts can yield innovative solutions that enhance health literacy and facilitate greater collaboration between experts and the public.

Education and awareness campaigns play a vital role in building bridges between experts and communities. Public health initiatives can focus on enhancing health literacy, emphasizing the importance of critical evaluation of health claims, particularly in discussions around alternative treatments like apricot seeds. These campaigns should involve multidisciplinary collaboration—drawing on insights from healthcare practitioners, health educators, and community leaders—to create comprehensive resources that address individual needs. Workshops, seminars, and online webinars can engage diverse audiences, promoting an understanding of risks and the importance of evidence-based choices.

Another crucial aspect of bridging gaps is acknowledging and respecting cultural beliefs surrounding health. Individuals often turn to alternative remedies due to cultural heritage or personal values. Experts must remain sensitive to these perspectives while facilitating dialogues that also emphasize safety and efficacy. By incorporating cultural understanding into health communication, we can engage communities meaningfully and ensure that discussions surrounding alternative treatments are respectful, evidence-based, and centered around patient well-being.

It is also essential to address the barriers that may impede communication between experts and the public. Trust may be eroded by perceived elitism or lack of empathy from healthcare professionals. Fostering relationships built on mutual respect and understanding is key to bridging these gaps. Listening to individuals' concerns, validating their experiences, and providing compassionate care can help restore trust, allowing for more fruitful discussions surrounding health choices.

Ultimately, bridging gaps between experts and the public is an intricate, multifaceted process that demands concerted efforts from all stakeholders involved in healthcare. By promoting transparency, utilizing accessible language, leveraging technology, fostering education and awareness, recognizing cultural beliefs, and prioritizing compassion, we can create a more informed public that navigates health choices wisely. As misinformation continues to threaten individual health decisions, particularly in the case of unverified treatments like apricot seeds, the importance of strong bridges between healthcare professionals and communities cannot be overstated. Through collective efforts, we can work toward a healthier society where informed choices prevail.

13. Spotlight on Health Communication in the Digital Age

13.1. The Evolution of Health Communication

The evolution of health communication has undergone significant transformations over the past few decades, particularly with the advent of digital technologies and the proliferation of information through the internet and social media. This evolution reflects a broader shift in how health-related information is produced, disseminated, and received by the public. It encompasses a wide range of strategies, practices, and challenges that impact the effectiveness of health campaigns, the engagement of diverse audiences, and the overall comprehension of critical health issues, including the contentious narrative surrounding alternative treatments such as apricot seeds for cancer.

Historically, health communication was largely one-directional, with medical professionals and institutions serving as the primary sources of information. Patients were often passive recipients of medical advice, with little opportunity for engagement or feedback. However, as medical knowledge expanded and the complexity of health issues grew, it became increasingly clear that effective communication is a multi-faceted endeavor. The recognition that patients needed to be informed, engaged, and empowered in their own health decisions led to the development of more interactive communication strategies.

The digital age introduced a paradigm shift in health communication. With the emergence of the internet, individuals gained access to a wealth of health information at their fingertips. Online resources, health websites, and social media platforms democratized health knowledge, allowing laypeople to engage in health discussions and share personal narratives. As a result, health communication is now characterized by a participatory approach, where individuals actively seek information, express their opinions, and share their experiences —dynamics that are particularly evident in conversations about alternative remedies like apricot seeds.

This shift, however, comes with its own set of challenges. The overwhelming volume of information available online can lead to confusion, as individuals are often confronted with conflicting claims and anecdotal evidence that lack scientific validation. The distinction between credible health information and misinformation is not always clear, particularly in the face of sensationalized health narratives that may prioritize emotional resonance over empirical evidence. The narrative surrounding apricot seeds as a potential cancer cure exemplifies this challenge, as anecdotal success stories can overshadow the critical evidence presented by the scientific community that categorically rejects unverified health claims.

Developing effective health campaigns in this complex landscape necessitates a deep understanding of target audiences and their values, beliefs, and motivations. To create compelling campaigns, health communicators must not only present accurate information but also resonate with individuals on an emotional level. By tailoring messaging to address the specific concerns and aspirations of diverse audiences, campaigns can foster trust and facilitate engagement. For instance, campaigns that highlight the risks associated with apricot seeds and provide evidence-based alternatives can empower individuals to make informed choices while acknowledging their emotions and desire for hope.

Leveraging digital platforms for health promotion involves the strategic use of social media, websites, apps, and online communities to disseminate health information and engage with the public. This approach allows for real-time communication and feedback, empowering individuals to share their experiences while cultivating a sense of community. However, digital platforms also present challenges, as misinformation can spread rapidly and reach vulnerable populations. Health communicators must strike a balance between utilizing these platforms to promote accurate information while actively countering false claims and sensationalized narratives.

Reaching diverse audiences poses another significant challenge in health communication. Various cultural, socioeconomic, and linguistic factors can influence how health messages are received and understood. To effectively communicate with diverse populations, health campaigns must adopt culturally competent approaches that center the experiences and values of different communities. In the case of alternative treatments, understanding the cultural significance of certain remedies is essential for fostering trust and facilitating conversations about evidence-based practices.

Collaboration with tech experts can enhance health communication efforts by providing innovative solutions that bridge gaps in public understanding. Developing user-friendly digital tools that ensure accessibility and accuracy of health information can empower individuals to navigate the complexities of their health journeys. Technology can enable health professionals to gather data on public perceptions, track misinformation trends, and tailor communication strategies accordingly, ultimately improving health literacy and patient outcomes.

As we analyze case studies in health communication, we recognize that lessons learned from past efforts can inform future strategies. For instance, understanding the failures of campaigns that relied on sensationalism rather than factual accuracy provides valuable insights into the importance of credibility in health communication. Similarly, campaigns that successfully integrated both traditional and digital methods offer guidance on how to engage diverse populations effectively.

In conclusion, the evolution of health communication reflects the shifting dynamics of how information is created, shared, and perceived in an increasingly digital world. The challenges posed by misinformation, emotional engagement, and the need for culturally competent approaches necessitate a commitment to thoughtful, evidence-based communication strategies that prioritize the well-being of individuals. By harnessing the power of digital platforms while remaining vigilant against the spread of false information, health communicators can foster a more informed public, enabling individuals to navigate their health choices wisely and safely.

13.2. Developing Effective Health Campaigns

In the evolving world of health communication, the importance of developing effective health campaigns cannot be overstated, especially when addressing the pervasive issue of misinformation about alternative treatments like apricot seeds purported to treat cancer. These campaigns are essential tools for shaping public perception, informing health choices, and ultimately promoting wellness. A well-crafted health campaign serves not only to disseminate accurate information but also to engage individuals on an emotional and intellectual level, fostering a sense of community and shared responsibility.

To begin with, the foundational principle of any effective health campaign is rooted in evidence-based information. Campaigns must be informed by the latest scientific research and public health guidelines. This involves not just presenting information but contextualizing it in a way that resonates with the target audience. For instance, a campaign addressing the risks associated with apricot seeds might provide clear and compelling data about their potential dangers, such as cyanide poisoning, while juxtaposing it against scientifically validated treatment alternatives. By clearly outlining the risks versus benefits, campaigns empower individuals to make informed choices regarding their health.

Leveraging digital platforms is one of the most impactful strategies in modern health campaigns. The ubiquitous presence of social media allows for the rapid dissemination of information, enabling health messages to reach wider audiences than ever before. Campaigns can utilize various formats, such as videos, infographics, and interactive posts, to engage users effectively and encourage sharing. By creating easily digestible content that is informative yet compelling, campaigns can capitalize on the viral nature of social media to combat misinformation and promote evidence-based alternatives.

However, challenges invariably arise in reaching diverse audiences. A successful health campaign must consider the cultural, linguistic, and socioeconomic backgrounds of its target audience. Tailoring messages to reflect the values and beliefs of different communities is essential. For example, campaigns addressing the use of apricot seeds should be sensitive to cultural traditions surrounding natural remedies while providing factual information that encourages critical thinking. Collaboration with community leaders and local organizations can amplify the campaign's reach and effectiveness, ensuring that the messaging resonates with the intended audience.

The role of collaborating with tech experts cannot be overlooked in the development of effective health campaigns. Engaging technology professionals to create user-friendly platforms or apps can facilitate easier access to credible health information. These tools can help individuals navigate the complexities of health choices, allowing them to evaluate claims critically and seek out evidence-based practices. By harnessing technology's capabilities, health campaigns can foster a more informed public while promoting proactive health behaviors.

An examination of case studies reveals valuable lessons in effective health communication. For instance, analyzing the failures of alternative treatments to gain traction can illuminate the dangers of sensationalized messaging without scientific backing. On the contrary, success stories from integrative approaches showcase the potential for collaboration between conventional and alternative methods when rooted in scientific evidence. These insights guide future campaign development, illustrating the importance of a multifaceted approach to health communication.

Moving forward, the emphasis on building knowledge through reliable sources is vital. Campaigns should encourage the exploration of credible scientific journals and resources that provide evidence-based information. Educating individuals on how to identify scientific consensus, leverage digital archives, and utilize technology to access credible health information can empower them to make informed health decisions. By fostering an environment of knowledge and responsibility, health campaigns can counteract the harms of misinformation effectively.

In conclusion, developing effective health campaigns is essential in the fight against misinformation surrounding alternative treatments. By prioritizing evidence-based information, leveraging digital platforms, adapting to diverse audiences, collaborating with technology experts, and emphasizing the importance of reliable sources, health campaigns can empower individuals to make informed choices. As we reflect on the evolving landscape of health communication, the commitment to fostering clear, accurate messaging and open dialogue between experts and the public can lead to healthier outcomes and improved community well-being. By navigating the complexities of health narratives, we can champion informed decision-making and ensure a safer, more empowered public in the quest for lifelong wellness.

13.3. Leveraging Digital Platforms for Health Promotion

In today's health landscape, the intersection of technology and communication has fundamentally transformed how information is disseminated and consumed. The advent of digital platforms has created unprecedented opportunities for health promotion, making it easier than ever for individuals to access information on various health topics, including information about alternative treatments like apricot seeds purported to treat cancer. However, the very benefits of these platforms also present a myriad of challenges, including the spread of misinformation and the difficulty in reaching diverse audiences.

When considering how to leverage digital platforms for health promotion, it is imperative to understand the importance of using evidence-based information. Individuals often turn to online sources for health advice, which means healthcare providers and public health organizations must actively participate in digital discussions to counteract the spread of unverified claims. The appeal of natural remedies, often fueled by emotional narratives and personal testimonials, can distract from scientific evidence. Thus, health communication must be clear, credible, and rooted in validated research.

Engaging with social media allows for rapid dissemination of accurate health information. Campaigns that utilize videos, visuals, and interactive content can effectively capture attention and communicate key messages about the risks of unverified treatments while offering evidence-based alternatives. For instance, using social media platforms to clearly outline the dangers of cyanide poisoning associated with apricot seeds, alongside promoting effective, scientifically-supported cancer treatments, is paramount in reshaping public perception around such remedies.

However, reaching diverse audiences remains a concern for health promotion efforts. Access to health information is not uniform, with inequities in healthcare access, literacy rates, and cultural perceptions influencing how various populations engage with health communications. Campaigns must therefore prioritize inclusivity, ensuring that content is culturally sensitive and resonates with different communities. By collaborating with community organizations and stakeholder groups, health communicators can develop strategies tailored to the unique needs of specific populations, ultimately increasing the efficacy of health promotion efforts.

Collaboration with technology experts can further enhance health promotion strategies. By creating user-friendly apps or websites that provide reliable health information, these partnerships can facilitate access to credible resources—empowering individuals to make informed decisions about their health. For example, technology can drive initiatives that allow users to verify health claims, track their well-being, and access expert guidance on alternative treatments.

Moreover, case studies from real-life scenarios can offer invaluable insights into successful health promotion strategies and highlight lessons learned from failures. For instance, analyzing the consequences of the promotion of apricot seeds reveals the critical need for accurate information, while case studies showcasing successful integrative approaches to treatment can highlight the benefits of collaborative medical practices that blend conventional and alternative medicine grounded in evidence.

As digital platforms continue to evolve, the need for continuous evaluation and adaptation of health promotion strategies becomes increasingly urgent. Innovations in medicine and technology provide opportunities to discover new ways to engage audiences and disseminate credible health information effectively. Advocacy for policies that support health literacy education and increased access to reliable resources can advance the health promotion agenda.

In conclusion, leveraging digital platforms for health promotion requires a multifaceted approach that incorporates evidence-based information, engagement with diverse audiences, and collaboration with technology experts. By fostering a commitment to clear communication, inclusivity, and adaptability, health promotion efforts can counterbalance misinformation while guiding individuals toward wise health choices that prioritize safety and well-being. The ongoing endeavor to improve public understanding of health topics will ultimately lead to healthier communities, where informed choices are championed, and the pursuit of wellness is recognized as a shared responsibility.

13.4. Challenges in Reaching Diverse Audiences

In reaching diverse audiences, particularly in health communication, several critical challenges emerge that require careful consideration and strategic planning. The narrative surrounding alternative treatments—like the promotion of apricot seeds as a potential cancer cure—serves as an illustrative example of the complexities involved in effectively engaging various demographic populations. Navigating these challenges requires an understanding of cultural differences, communication barriers, and the dynamic nature of health beliefs.

One major challenge lies in the way cultural perceptions of health and wellness intersect with individual experiences. Different cultural backgrounds bring diverse beliefs about the efficacy of natural remedies versus conventional medical approaches. For example, in some communities, traditional herbal medicine holds significant credence and trust as an integral part of health-care practices. In such cases, health communicators must respect these cultural values while simultaneously presenting factual evidence regarding the risks of unverified treatments like apricot seeds. This requires a nuanced approach that honors cultural perspectives while encouraging a dialogue grounded in scientific evidence.

Communication barriers can also complicate efforts to reach diverse audiences. Language differences and varying levels of health literacy across populations can hinder effective engagement. For instance, individuals who may not be proficient in the language of the health information being communicated might struggle to understand nuanced risks surrounding a treatment. As health campaigns strive to reach broader audiences, producing materials in multiple languages and employing culturally relevant imagery can enhance accessibility and comprehension. It is essential for health communication strategies to ensure that messages resonate with varying literacy levels while addressing potential misunderstandings.

Additionally, the challenge of misinformation can disproportionately affect marginalized communities. Due to historical distrust in the medical system and health authorities, individuals from these populations may turn to alternative sources of information, which may lack credibility. This underscores the importance of building trust through transparency and community engagement. Health communicators should establish relationships with local leaders and organizations to facilitate dialogues and actively listen to the concerns and experiences of the community. Creating a network of trusted voices can serve as a conduit for accurate health information and promote responsible public health messaging.

The digital landscape presents both opportunities and challenges in reaching diverse audiences as well. Digital platforms allow for the rapid dissemination of health information, but they can also be a double-edged sword in terms of exposing individuals to misinformation. Online health narratives surrounding apricot seeds may be compelling; however, they often amplify sensational claims without sufficient scrutiny. To counteract this effect, health organizations must develop digital literacy campaigns that empower individuals to critically evaluate the information they encounter. This involves training people to question the validity of claims, check sources, and seek evidence-based health information.

Moreover, public health initiatives must emphasize inclusivity and diversifying narratives that represent various perspectives and experiences. Campaigns should highlight stories from individuals within different cultural groups who have successfully navigated their health journeys, whether through conventional treatments or integrative approaches. Sharing diverse experiences fosters community connection, increases the relatability of the message, and helps counter isolation that some individuals may feel when confronting health challenges.

Finally, collaboration with specialists and community stakeholders is paramount in overcoming the challenges of reaching diverse audiences. Working closely with cultural consultants, healthcare providers, and local organizations allows for the development of tailored outreach strategies that encompass the needs and beliefs of specific populations. By involving various stakeholders in the planning and execution of health communication efforts, public health campaigns can enhance their efficacy, promote trust, and foster a culture of informed health choices.

In conclusion, the challenges in reaching diverse audiences in health communication require multifaceted solutions centered on cultural sensitivity, improved accessibility, and the fostering of trust. By recognizing these challenges and developing strategic approaches to address them, health communicators can meaningfully engage with diverse populations, ensuring that effective, evidence-based information reaches those who most need it. This, in turn, can help mitigate the risks posed by alternative treatments and empower individuals to make informed decisions about their health.

13.5. Collaborating with Tech Experts for Better Outcomes

In today's rapidly evolving health landscape, collaboration with tech experts can play a transformative role in enhancing health outcomes and addressing misinformation, particularly concerning alternative treatments such as apricot seeds touted as cancer cures. The integration of technology into health communication not only increases the accessibility of accurate information but also empowers individuals to make informed choices regarding their health. This subchapter will explore various pathways through which healthcare professionals and tech experts can work together to amplify health messages, mitigate risks associated with misinformation, and ultimately improve health literacy.

One of the primary ways tech experts can contribute to health outcomes is through the development of health-focused applications and platforms. These technologies can provide users with access to reliable health information, facilitate self-monitoring of health conditions, and bolster engagement in preventive care. For example, applications designed to educate users about the risks associated with unverified treatments, including apricot seeds, can empower individuals to critically assess health claims and seek evidence-based alternatives. By leveraging features such as push notifications, interactive quizzes, and personalized health recommendations, these applications can effectively foster a culture of informed health decision-making.

Moreover, the role of social media in health communication cannot be understated. Collaborating with tech experts to create engaging campaigns that disseminate accurate health messaging on platforms that reach diverse audiences can significantly counteract the influx of misinformation. For instance, developing shareable graphics or concise videos focused on the risks associated with apricot seeds can capture attention and circulate rapidly, allowing health organizations to reclaim the narrative and present a fact-based perspective. Social media analytics can also provide valuable insights into public perceptions and misinformation trends, enabling ongoing refinement of communication strategies.

Furthermore, the use of data analytics stands to enhance health communication efforts by identifying trends in public inquiries and health behaviors. For instance, analyzing search queries and social media interactions regarding apricot seeds can shed light on the extent of misinformation in circulation. By collaborating with data scientists, healthcare organizations can develop targeted communication strategies that address misconceptions directly and educate the public about evidence-based alternatives. This data-driven approach empowers health professionals to proactively engage with communities and provide guidance on safe treatment options.

Open-source platforms are another avenue for collaboration between healthcare professionals and tech experts. Creating user-friendly databases that compile trustworthy health information can serve as a valuable resource for individuals seeking credible insights into various treatments. These platforms can facilitate discussion forums where users can engage with health professionals, seek advice, and share experiences without the distortions often associated with unverified health claims. By promoting transparency and community engagement, these open-source initiatives empower individuals to critically analyze the information they receive while fostering an environment ripe for informed discussion.

In addition to technological advancements, prioritizing digital health literacy is crucial in fostering informed health choices. Tech experts can collaborate with public health organizations to develop educational resources that empower individuals to discern credible sources and evaluate health claims critically. Workshops, webinars, and online courses can enhance digital literacy skills, enabling individuals to navigate the complexities of health information effectively. For example, providing step-by-step guidance on how to assess the credibility of claims surrounding apricot seeds will facilitate more responsible decision-making.

Moreover, addressing the emotional aspects of health decision-making is essential when collaborating with tech experts. Individuals seeking alternative remedies often grapple with fear and uncertainty, leading them to seek solace in online narratives that promote hope. By leveraging technology to provide compassionate care through telehealth services, virtual support groups, and guided mindfulness exercises, healthcare professionals can build rapport with patients, helping them to feel more empowered while also conveying critical safety information regarding unvalidated remedies.

Finally, reinforcing the importance of a multifaceted approach in health communication will arise from collaboration with tech experts. The complexities of health narratives surrounding alternative treatments necessitate a comprehensive strategy that embraces the strengths of both healthcare professionals and technology. Creating repositories of accurate health information, promoting digital health literacy, and employing technology to disseminate educational resources can enhance the public's capacity to make informed decisions regarding their health.

In conclusion, collaborating with tech experts to leverage the advantages of digital tools and platforms represents a promising pathway to improve health outcomes and combat misinformation. Through innovative technologies, data analytics, open-source platforms, and education initiatives, stakeholders can foster an environment of informed decision-making, particularly concerning alternative treatments like apricot seeds. By prioritizing health literacy and addressing the emotional aspects of treatment choices, the collaborative efforts of healthcare professionals and tech experts can cultivate a culture of safety, empowerment, and evidence-based health practices. As we navigate the complexities of health communication, embracing technology as a partner can lead us toward a healthier, more informed society.

14. Case Studies: Lessons From Real-Life Scenarios

14.1. Analyzing Alternative Treatment Failures

In the quest to understand and critically analyze alternative treatment failures, it is essential to explore multiple facets, including the context within which these treatments arise, the social and psychological factors that influence their popularity, and the impacts of misinformation. This investigation sheds light on the broader implications of health narratives, particularly when misguided beliefs about remedies like apricot seeds for cancer capture public enthusiasm without the backing of scientific evidence.

Understanding the allure of alternative treatments begins with recognizing that many of these solutions emerge from a desire for agency in health decisions—that innate human urge to reclaim control in the face of life-threatening illnesses. In an environment where conventional medical treatments can feel impersonal and fraught with complications, patients often search for answers that resonate with their emotions and cultural beliefs. Alternative remedies, often portrayed as simple, natural solutions, can fulfill this need, even in the absence of solid empirical support.

The case of apricot seeds exemplifies this dynamic. Advocates of apricot seeds claim that the compounds within them can combat cancerous cells—claims that have gained traction largely through anecdotal evidence rather than rigorous scientific validation. The notion that something as humble as a seed could yield such profound healing resonates deeply with individuals grappling with the uncertainty of cancer diagnoses. However, this compelling narrative often overshadows the significant health risks associated with the consumption of apricot seeds, primarily due to their amygdalin content, which can metabolize into toxic cyanide.

Analyzing these alternative treatment failures informs our understanding of the consequences of misinformation. Historical examples highlight the blatant risks individuals face when they forego evi-

164

dence-based practices in favor of unverified remedies. The laetrile movement in the mid-20th century, largely centered around claims of apricot kernels as cancer cures, serves as a stark reminder of how desperation can lead patients to embrace dangerous alternatives. The subsequent surge in cases of cyanide poisoning associated with laetrile usage illuminates the critical necessity for rigorous scientific inquiry before accepting health claims as valid.

Equally significant are the social dynamics that perpetuate alternative treatment narratives. Personal success stories circulate widely in online communities, often presented as definitive proof of efficacy. These compelling testimonials can elicit emotional responses that reinforce beliefs in the healing power of unverified remedies, leading patients to ignore substantial scientific evidence to the contrary. The psychological draw of these narratives showcases the challenge of separating emotional appeals from factual realities, underscoring the need for better education and communication surrounding health choices.

Furthermore, the role of healthcare professionals and public health advocates becomes paramount in challenging established narratives surrounding alternative treatments. By actively engaging with patients and providing clear, evidence-based information, providers can counter misleading claims and promote responsible health choices. This requires a commitment to transparency, education, and the establishment of trust within patient-provider relationships.

Understanding the nuances surrounding alternative treatment failures also extends to the need for policymakers to create safeguards against the marketing of unverified remedies. Regulatory oversight becomes necessary to protect the public from dangerous claims made by individuals or entities promoting alternative treatments without adequate scientific backing. Striking a balance between health freedom and consumer protection becomes critical, ensuring that individuals are aware of the risks associated with unregulated practices while still preserving their right to explore alternative options.

The analysis of alternative treatment failures ultimately underlines the importance of evidence-based health communication. By informing individuals about the inherent risks of unverified alternatives, fostering critical thinking skills, and promoting health literacy, we can empower patients to make informed decisions about their health. The story of apricot seeds and similar alternatives should serve as a guide—a transparent call for health advocacy that prioritizes safety, efficacy, and informed choice above sensationalized narratives.

Understanding these dynamics informs the broader conversation on health choices—encouraging us to remain vigilant against misinformation while fostering a culture of inquiry and evidence-based decision-making. As we navigate the complexities of health and wellness, it is through these reflections that we can promote wiser, safer health choices that prioritize the well-being of all individuals. By focusing on education and critical engagement, we can foster a community dedicated to informed health decisions that embrace the full spectrum of both traditional and alternative practices grounded in rigorous scientific support.

Ultimately, the exploration of alternative treatment failures encourages a more nuanced understanding of health narratives, one that values knowledge, empowers individuals, and rebukes the myths that often lead to harmful choices. Through continued dialogue, advocacy, and the promotion of evidence-based practices, we can foster healthier communities where choices reflect both autonomy and informed insight, paving the way for a future founded on well-being.

14.2. Successes of Integrative Approaches

In today's rapidly evolving health landscape, the successes of integrative approaches, particularly in the context of alternative treatments such as apricot seeds for cancer, highlight the importance of combining traditional health practices with modern medical insights. Integrative medicine emphasizes not only the use of conventional therapies but also the consideration of holistic and patient-centered approaches. This subchapter will explore the successes of integrative medicine, examining how different modalities, when combined effectively, can lead to enhanced patient outcomes and a more comprehensive framework for care.

One pivotal success of integrative approaches is their emphasis on treating the whole person rather than merely addressing symptoms or diseases in isolation. For example, when individuals are diagnosed with cancer, their physical health is often accompanied by emotional, psychological, and social challenges. Integrative medicine recognizes the interconnected nature of these aspects and fosters treatment plans that address not only the disease but also the well-being of the patient in a holistic manner. This can involve incorporating therapies such as acupuncture, massage, nutrition counseling, and mindfulness practices alongside conventional treatments like chemotherapy or radiation. The result is a more rounded care experience that can alleviate anxiety and improve overall quality of life, which is intrinsically valuable, particularly for patients facing the rigors of cancer treatment.

Research supporting the efficacy of integrative approaches has expanded significantly, demonstrating positive outcomes ranging from improved pain management to enhanced emotional resilience. Studies have shown that patients who participate in integrative therapies often report lower levels of stress and anxiety, improved coping strategies, and a greater sense of control over their health. This is particularly relevant in the context of discussions around alternatives like apricot seeds; while the seeds may evoke emotional responses tied to simplicity and natural healing, the integrative framework encourages patients to evaluate various options holistically. It promotes the idea of informed decision-making rather than merely adhering to singular, unverified methods.

Another success of integrative medicine is its adaptability to diverse patient needs and preferences. By recognizing that each individual may respond differently to treatment modalities, integrative approaches allow for a customizable framework that respects personal choices. This is especially important in the discussions surrounding natural remedies such as apricot seeds, where some patients may feel a cultural or personal connection to natural healing practices. Integrative medicine gives patients the agency to explore these options while ensuring they remain grounded in evidence-based practices.

Furthermore, integrative approaches facilitate collaboration between various healthcare providers, emphasizing interdisciplinary communication among oncologists, nutritionists, therapists, and alternative health practitioners. This teamwork can enhance the continuum of care and ensure that patients receive cohesive support. For instance, while a medical doctor may suggest conventional treatments, a nutritionist can provide dietary guidance that complements these practices, and a therapist can assist with the psychological impacts of a cancer diagnosis. This holistic collaboration ultimately results in improved adherence to treatment plans and, consequently, better patient outcomes.

The success of integrative practices can also be observed in clinical settings that have embraced these principles. Hospitals and cancer treatment centers around the globe are increasingly incorporating integrative medicine programs designed to provide complementary therapies alongside standard oncological care. These programs often lead to higher patient satisfaction rates and decreased symptom burden, further reinforcing the value of well-rounded health strategies.

Still, implementing integrative approaches does not come without its challenges. While there is growing evidence supporting the effectiveness of certain complementary therapies, the need for further research and validation is essential. Establishing a clear scientific basis for these therapies ensures that patients can make informed decisions while minimizing the risk of harmful or ineffective treatments. It is vital to advocate for continued funding of research into integrative modalities and their outcomes to enhance our understanding of how these practices can synergize with conventional care.

As we reflect on the successes of integrative approaches, it becomes clear that a harmonious blend of traditional medicine and alternative therapies holds great promise for the future of healthcare. By prioritizing patient-centered care, respecting individuals' health beliefs, and fostering interdisciplinary collaboration, practitioners can create a more inclusive and effective healthcare environment.

In conclusion, the exploration of integrative approaches highlights the importance of fostering health strategies that honor both the complexities of the human experience and the necessity for informed decision-making. In navigating choices surrounding alternative treatments like apricot seeds, a balanced perspective rooted in integrative principles can empower individuals, ensuring they receive holistic care that prioritizes their overall well-being and enhances their quality of life as they engage in their health journeys.

14.3. Impacts of Policy in Different Regions

In different regions around the world, the impacts of policies related to health, particularly those concerning the regulation of alternative treatments like apricot seeds, can vary significantly. These regional differences are shaped by cultural beliefs, healthcare systems, and the regulatory environment that governs health practices. Understanding these impacts is crucial for comprehending how misinformation can spread and how effective public health interventions can be implemented.

In some regions, particularly in the West, rigorous clinical trials and scientific research underpin the approval and promotion of medical treatments. Policymaking in these areas often emphasizes evidence-based approaches, focusing on the importance of regulatory oversight to ensure patient safety. The U.S. Food and Drug Administration (FDA), for example, has firmly asserted its stance on apricot seeds, clearly outlining the risks associated with their consumption due to the presence of cyanogenic compounds that can lead to cyanide poisoning. In this regulatory environment, marketing unverified health claims, especially those promising miraculous cures, faces stringent scrutiny. Public health campaigns in these regions strive to educate individuals on the scientifically supported treatments and the potential dangers of alternative remedies, thereby fostering a more informed public.

Conversely, in many developing regions, the context surrounding health treatments can be markedly different. In areas where access to conventional healthcare is limited, individuals may increasingly turn to alternative treatments, including natural remedies deeply entrenched in cultural practices. The efficacy of these treatments is often based on anecdotal evidence and traditional knowledge, which may not always be supported by scientific validation. In such environments, apricot seeds and similar remedies may be celebrated as part of cultural health practices, with less regulatory scrutiny regarding their safety or effectiveness. Consequently, the health policies governing these regions may focus more on integrating traditional practices within broader healthcare frameworks rather than challenging their efficacy based on scientific evidence.

The influence of local beliefs and practices can shape how policy impacts public perception of treatments. In regions where there is a strong belief in the healing properties of natural remedies, public trust in scientifically unverified claims can overshadow concerns about their safety. Health policies may, therefore, encounter resistance when attempting to promote information about the risks associated with these remedies, leading to a complex dynamic between governmental health messages and individual beliefs.

Furthermore, the global accessibility of information through the internet adds another layer of complexity. Misinformation related to alternative treatments can propagate rapidly across borders, irrespective of the regulatory measures in place. Social media campaigns promoting apricot seeds as a natural cancer cure may reach audiences in various regions, fueling public interest and potentially leading individuals to adopt these remedies without understanding the associated risks. The challenge arises when local health policies fail to keep pace with the rapid spread of misinformation, which can lead to public health crises stemming from the adverse effects of unverified treatments.

Regional differences in healthcare literacy further amplify these challenges. In some populations, individuals may lack the resources or understanding necessary to critically evaluate health claims, making them more susceptible to believing in the efficacy of unproven remedies like apricot seeds. Health education campaigns must, therefore, be tailored to address these disparities, ensuring that all groups have access to accurate and reliable information regarding health treatments.

Moreover, addressing the impacts of health policies and regulations necessitates a global viewpoint that embraces collaboration between regions. Sharing best practices, and insights, and allowing for the exchange of information on effective public health interventions can contribute to stronger global health responses. This approach can be particularly effective in disseminating accurate information about risks associated with alternative treatments, encouraging the promotion of evidence-based practices that prioritize patient safety and well-being.

In conclusion, the impacts of policy on health practices regarding alternative treatments like apricot seeds are shaped by various factors, including cultural beliefs, healthcare systems, and regulatory environments. Understanding these regional differences is vital for developing effective public health interventions that can combat misinformation and promote safe health choices. By addressing health literacy, fostering informed discussions, and celebrating the integration of traditional practices within safe frameworks, we can work towards a more comprehensive understanding of health that respects individual beliefs while emphasizing the importance of scientific evidence.

14.4. Learning from Survivor Narratives

Learning from survivor narratives yields valuable insights into the intertwining of personal experience, health beliefs, and the ways in which these components can shape public discourse about alternative remedies. This approach emphasizes the importance of storytelling in health communication, particularly as narratives from individuals diagnosed with cancer can highlight the emotional complexities associated with treatment choices, including the appeal of unverified options such as apricot seeds.

Survivor narratives play a critical role in the health landscape by giving voice to the experiences of individuals who have navigated their health journeys. These stories often capture the raw emotions, struggles, and triumphs faced by patients, underscoring the psychological and social dimensions of illness. When individuals share their encounters with traditional and alternative treatments, such narratives can create a rich tapestry of understanding around health choices, touching on vulnerability, hope, and resilience. For those grappling with serious illnesses, these testimonials can serve as sources of inspiration or caution.

However, it is crucial to approach survivor narratives critically. While personal experiences can offer valuable insights, they should not be misconstrued as definitive evidence. The passion and emotion shared in survivor stories about the use of apricot seeds can evoke strong emotional responses, but they should also be contextualized within a framework that acknowledges the lack of scientific validation for such claims. This disparity highlights the need for balanced communication that respects individual experiences while prioritizing the rigors of empirical evidence.

Navigating the complexities of survivor narratives requires mindful engagement from health professionals and advocates. Listening to the stories and perspectives of patients provides opportunities to foster trust and empathy, creating rapport that can pave the way for meaningful health discussions. By acknowledging the emotional weight of survivor narratives, practitioners can foster open dialogue about the risks and benefits of both conventional and complementary treatments, encouraging patients to explore their health choices responsibly.

Moreover, survivor narratives can serve as catalysts for broader public health discussions. When shared within community forums, health campaigns, or social media platforms, these voices can bring visibility to issues surrounding alternative remedies and encourage critical reflection on unverified claims. For instance, highlighting survivor experiences in the context of apricot seeds can prompt discussions about the emotional allure of natural treatments, while also emphasizing the importance of informed decision-making based on scientific consensus.

The potential pitfalls of survivor narratives must also be addressed. As individuals share their stories, they may unintentionally promote unverified claims regarding treatments that lack scientific backing. In doing so, there is a risk of reinforcing the notion that personal experiences are sufficient evidence to validate health claims, particularly when it comes to dangerous alternatives like apricot seeds. Education initiatives should emphasize that while survivor stories are impactful, they cannot replace the critical need for empirical research and consensus among health experts.

To harness the power of survivor narratives effectively, health communicators should consider integrating these stories into evidence-based health campaigns. By framing narratives within a context that respects both lived experience and scientific inquiry, advocates can leverage the emotional resonance of survivor stories while reinforcing the importance of safe health practices. This balance can foster a community dialogue that prioritizes safety, empowerment, and responsible health choices.

In conclusion, learning from survivor narratives offers a rich resource for understanding the emotional complexities surrounding health decisions, particularly in relation to alternative treatments like apricot seeds. Engaging with these stories provides opportunities for empathy, education, and advocacy. However, it is imperative to honor the complexities of personal experiences while grounding discussions in scientific evidence to ensure that public health messages remain accurate and responsible. By carefully navigating the terrain of survivor narratives, we can foster a culture of informed choice and empower individuals to make health decisions that prioritize safety, efficacy, and well-being.

14.5. Future Directions in Treatment Research

As we step into the future of treatment research, it is essential to consider the evolving landscape of healthcare, where integrating scientific inquiry with patient-centered practices will play a vital role. The quest for effective treatments—intelligently designed through rigorous empirical studies—will continue to intersect with the growing emphasis on personalized healthcare. Within this framework, we will investigate key areas poised for innovation, the importance of nuanced public engagement, and the ongoing challenges posed by misinformation, particularly in the context of alternative therapies, exemplified by the narrative surrounding apricot seeds.

The first significant direction in treatment research is the drive toward personalized medicine, where therapies are tailored to the unique genetic makeup of patients and their specific health circumstances. As advancements in genomics continue at a rapid pace, researchers will likely develop targeted therapies that more effectively address the molecular characteristics of individual tumors. The promise of precision oncology holds the potential to revolutionize cancer treatment, presenting options that go beyond traditional modalities and resonating with patients who seek control over their treatment paths. However, the financial implications and accessibility of these therapies remain critical challenges that must be addressed to ensure equitable access for all populations.

Emerging technologies will also revolutionize treatment research and delivery in the coming years. For instance, artificial intelligence and machine learning are gradually being integrated into healthcare, providing researchers with sophisticated tools to analyze vast datasets and identify patterns that can inform treatment pathways. The ability to predict individual responses to therapies through data analytics could profoundly impact decision-making processes and improve overall patient outcomes. However, building trust in these technologies and ensuring patient privacy will be vital as these tools gain traction in clinical research and practice.

In parallel, the integration of community health perspectives into treatment research is gaining recognition as an essential component of addressing health disparities. Engaging communities in discussions about their health needs and the appropriateness of specific treatments can foster participation and ensure that research addresses the social determinants of health that impact access and outcomes. This holistic approach will cultivate collaborative relationships between researchers, practitioners, and the public, amplifying efforts to develop relevant, effective interventions that resonate with diverse populations.

Furthermore, maintaining a focus on ethical considerations in treatment research is paramount. The narrative surrounding apricot seeds serves as a cautionary tale emphasizing the ethical obligation to educate patients about the risks of unverified treatments. As researchers strive for groundbreaking discoveries, they must continually evaluate the moral implications of their work, particularly when dealing with vulnerable populations. Safeguarding patient interests should remain at the forefront, ensuring that research prioritizes safety, informed consent, and transparency.

Moreover, attention to public health campaigns will be crucial in disseminating credible information and countering misinformation that proliferates in digital spaces. Through strategic health communication efforts, professionals can anticipate public reactions to new research findings, clarify misconceptions, and foster open dialogues between experts and communities. This proactive engagement presents an opportunity to reinforce the importance of evidence-based practices while respecting individuals' beliefs and values.

In considering the challenges of misinformation, harnessing the power of education across diverse populations remains paramount in shaping treatment narratives. Building health literacy initiatives that are culturally sensitive and accessible will empower individuals to evaluate health claims critically and advocate for their own well-being. Ensuring that patients can discern credible sources will fortify their ability to navigate the complexities of health information while promoting a culture of informed choices.

Additionally, the way in which scientific consensus is communicated will play a critical role in preparing for future health needs. The importance of bridging gaps between experts and the public by fostering collaboration in the discourse will shape adequately informed communities that can effectively digest new research findings and adapt their health practices accordingly. Educating the public on the processes behind scientific consensus will enhance understanding and acceptance of new treatments as they emerge, ensuring that innovations are met with enthusiasm rather than skepticism.

In conclusion, the future directions in treatment research present a promising yet complex landscape shaped by innovations in personalized medicine, technological advancements, ethical considerations, community engagement, and proactive communications. As we navigate this ever-evolving terrain, we must remain vigilant against misinformation, providing patients with the tools they need to evaluate alternative treatments critically. By fostering collaboration among researchers, healthcare practitioners, policymakers, and communities, we can build a robust and holistic approach to treatment research that acknowledges individual needs while prioritizing safety, efficacy, and informed decision-making. Together, we can aspire toward a future where health choices are not just informed but advocate for the well-being of every individual in the face of various health challenges.

15. Building Knowledge: A Guide to Reliable Sources

15.1. Identifying Credible Scientific Journals

Identifying credible scientific journals is a crucial step in the quest for reliable health information, especially in contexts rife with misinformation, such as the claims about apricot seeds as a treatment for cancer. A systematic evaluation of scientific sources enables individuals to access trustworthy research, empowering them to make informed health choices based on sound evidence.

When seeking credible scientific journals, there are several key criteria to consider. Firstly, it's imperative to assess whether the journal is peer-reviewed. Peer review is the process by which experts in the relevant field evaluate the manuscript before publication, ensuring that the research is rigorous, robust, and meets the journal's scholarly standards. Journals like "The New England Journal of Medicine," "The Journal of the American Medical Association (JAMA)," and "The Lancet" are renowned for their strict peer-review processes and are generally considered credible sources.

Another essential factor in evaluating journals is their impact factor, which measures the average number of citations to articles published within a specific timeframe. A higher impact factor often indicates that the journal's articles are well-regarded in the scientific community and frequently referenced by other researchers. However, it's important to recognize that impact factors should not be the only determinant of a journal's credibility, as some highly specialized journals may have lower impact factors despite publishing high-quality research.

The scope and subject relevance of the journal also play a pivotal role in determining its credibility. Specific journals focus on particular areas of health and medicine, meaning they will have researchers who specialize in those fields reviewing and publishing articles. For instance, when exploring claims related to apricot seeds and cancer treatment, journals dedicated to oncology, nutrition, or alternative medicine may be particularly relevant. Journals such as "Cancer Research," "Nutrition and Cancer," or "Complementary Therapies in Medicine" could provide insights into the efficacy and safety of alternative treatments.

A journal's affiliation with respected professional societies or academic institutions can further enhance its credibility. Many reputable journals are published by prominent medical associations, which helps ensure that they adhere to ethical publication standards and promote high-quality research. When assessing journals, look for those backed by organizations like the American Cancer Society or the National Institutes of Health, which lend additional authority to the research published therein.

In addition to these factors, it is also beneficial to examine the editorial board of the journal. An editorial board composed of recognized experts in the relevant fields adds credibility to the journal, as it reflects the level of scholarly oversight and commitment to maintaining publication integrity. Reviewing the credentials and affiliations of the members of the editorial board can provide insight into the quality and credibility of the research published in that journal.

Furthermore, accessing databases that index reputable journals is a helpful strategy in identifying credible sources. Databases such as PubMed, Scopus, and Web of Science are excellent resources that catalog scientific literature based on their quality and relevance. By relying on these databases, individuals can filter search results to find peer-reviewed articles, systematic reviews, and clinical trials that provide strong evidence for making health-informed decisions.

Lastly, individuals should be cautious about predatory journals—publications that lack peer review and editorial oversight but may still present themselves as credible. These journals often aim to profit from authors seeking to publish without adhering to rigorous academic standards. Common red flags include overwhelming fees for publication without a clear peer-review process, vague editorial policies, and a lack of indexing on reputable databases. Tools such as the Directory of Open Access Journals (DOAJ) can help identify legitimate open-access publications, ensuring that research is disseminated responsibly.

In conclusion, identifying credible scientific journals involves evaluating factors such as peer review, impact factor, subject relevance, affiliations, and editorial oversight. Relying on established databases can further enhance access to trustworthy research. By discerning credible sources, individuals can empower themselves with evidence-based information, enabling informed decisions regarding their health, particularly in navigating topics filled with misinformation, such as those surrounding apricot seeds and alternative cancer treatments. Through a commitment to critical evaluation of scientific literature, we can cultivate a more informed public discourse that prioritizes safety, efficacy, and wellness.

15.2. The Role of Libraries and Digital Archives

Libraries and digital archives play a vital role in the contemporary landscape of health information, serving as essential repositories of knowledge that empower individuals to make informed decisions about their health. In an era characterized by the rapid spread of information—much of which can be misleading or outright false—the necessity of reliable sources and credible documentation becomes increasingly paramount. This subchapter explores the significance of libraries and digital archives in providing access to trustworthy health information, particularly in relation to controversial claims surrounding alternative treatments like apricot seeds for cancer.

At the heart of libraries and digital archives is their commitment to preserving accurate knowledge and fostering health literacy. Libraries, by their very nature, curate collections that encompass a myriad of subjects, including comprehensive health information. This information includes scientific literature, research studies, and verified data from reputable sources—all of which are pivotal in empowering individuals to engage with their health actively. By offering access to academic journals, books, and reference materials, libraries serve as invaluable sanctuaries of knowledge where individuals can explore the complexities of health and well-being thoughtfully.

Digital archives expand upon this foundation, harnessing technology to facilitate broader access to health information. The increasing digitization of health-related literature means that individuals can retrieve research and resources from anywhere, at any time. This is particularly relevant when addressing the discourse surrounding alternative remedies, such as apricot seeds. When seeking to evaluate the claims about their efficacy, individuals can turn to digital archives housing peer-reviewed articles and empirical studies that rigorously assess the outcomes and risks associated with such claims, allowing them to navigate the topic effectively.

Moreover, health-focused libraries and digital archives provide essential support for health professionals, researchers, and public health advocates. The research conducted in these facilities informs evidence-based practices and public health policies, allowing professionals to rely on up-to-date information when making treatment recommendations or addressing public health crises. This proliferation of accurate information also bolsters advocacy efforts, ensuring that health campaigns are driven by credible data rather than individual anecdotes.

Libraries and digital archives also serve as educational resources. Workshops and programs organized by these institutions can empower community members with the skills they need to critically evaluate health information. Programs that teach health literacy in local libraries create opportunities for individuals to learn how to discern credible information from misinformation. By providing resources and guidance on how to navigate the ever-expanding digital landscape, libraries and archives help individuals cultivate a discerning approach to their health choices.

Another vital aspect of libraries and digital archives is their commitment to inclusivity. They play a crucial role in offering resources in multiple languages and accessible formats for diverse populations. As misinformation about alternative treatments often disproportionately affects marginalized communities, libraries can forge pathways for equitable access to reliable health information. This inclusivity fosters trust and encourages individuals to seek out credible sources instead of relying solely on anecdotal narratives that may lead them astray.

In addition, the collaborative partnerships that libraries and digital archives can establish with local health organizations, universities, and public health entities significantly enhance their capacity to provide accurate health information. These partnerships can streamline access to vital resources, ensuring that communities receive information that resonates with their unique needs while still relying on verified science.

As we look ahead, the evolution of libraries and digital archives will play a growing role in shaping health communication. The ability to synthesize vast amounts of information and present it in user-friendly formats positions these institutions as vital players in combating misinformation. Increasingly sophisticated digital tools, including artificial intelligence and machine learning algorithms, can optimize how individuals find and engage with health information, facilitating more informed decision-making.

In conclusion, libraries and digital archives serve as indispensable resources for health communication in a world characterized by information saturation. Through their dedication to curating reliable material, promoting health literacy, ensuring equitable access, and collaborating with community partners, these institutions empower individuals to make informed health choices—particularly in navigating the complexities surrounding alternative treatments like apricot seeds. As digital information grows more pervasive, the continued evolution and engagement of libraries and archives will be essential in championing a culture of evidence-based health understanding and fostering lifelong wellness in our communities.

15.3. Understanding Scientific Consensus

Understanding scientific consensus is a foundational aspect in the evolving discourse surrounding health claims, particularly in relation to alternative treatments like apricot seeds, which are often promoted as remedies for serious illnesses such as cancer. This subchapter seeks to demystify the concept of scientific consensus, exploring its importance in guiding health decisions, its formation process within the scientific community, and the implications of disregarding empirical research in favor of anecdotal evidence.

Scientific consensus refers to the collective agreement within the scientific community regarding specific conclusions based on the synthesis of substantial evidence gathered through rigorous research and peer-reviewed studies. This collective understanding does not emerge overnight; rather, it is the outcome of a prolonged process of inquiry, debate, and verification. The path to consensus typically encompasses the formulation of hypotheses, the design and execution of experimental studies, and the iterative challenge posed through peer review and critique.

In the realm of health and medicine, scientific consensus serves as an essential compass that directs clinical practice and public health policy. When discussing treatments such as apricot seeds, understanding the nature of scientific consensus is critical, particularly given the misleading narratives surrounding their supposed efficacy. While proponents of apricot seeds may share personal testimonials about their health benefits, these anecdotal claims stand in stark contrast to the broader scientific evidence available.

The process through which scientific consensus is established involves multiple stages of investigation, including systematic reviews and meta-analyses that aggregate findings across various studies. Researchers examine the quality of evidence, assess potential biases, and evaluate outcomes to arrive at a collective understanding. For instance, in the case of cancer treatments, robust scientific reviews have repeatedly demonstrated that claims surrounding the efficacy of apricot seeds lack substantial evidence and highlight the associated risks of cyanide toxicity. These rigorous evaluations reinforce the weight of scientific consensus—underscoring why health claims should be approached with caution.

However, the existence of scientific consensus presents a challenge in the face of misinformation. Many individuals often engage with health claims that resonate with their beliefs, frequently relying on personal anecdotes rather than confronting the available scientific research. This cognitive bias can lead individuals to outright reject the scientific consensus, favoring narratives that stem from emotional connections rather than evidence. The allure of narratives that present natural cures as efficacious solutions reflects underlying psychological needs—such as the desire for agency and simplicity in the face of complex health issues like cancer. As stories about apricot seeds circulate, they can overshadow rigorous scientific discourse, making it vital to reinforce the importance of scientific consensus in health decision-making.

Addressing the disconnect between personal beliefs and scientific consensus requires proactive health communication initiatives. Public health authorities and healthcare professionals must strive to disseminate reliable information that emphasizes the importance of scientific evidence while conversing with individuals about their personal beliefs. Both sides of the discourse should facilitate open dialogue, fostering space where individuals feel heard while simultaneously receiving information grounded in empirical research.

Additionally, educating the public about the nature of scientific inquiry and the consensus-building process is paramount for enhancing health literacy. Initiatives that teach critical thinking skills enable individuals to navigate health discussions more effectively and assess the credibility of claims they encounter. Such education empowers individuals to approach health decisions with skepticism and care, ultimately enhancing their ability to discern fact from fiction.

The role of researchers also remains crucial in upholding scientific consensus against the tide of misleading health claims. Building public trust in the scientific community entails transparent communication of research findings, fostering dialogue between scientists and the communities they serve. By actively engaging in discussions about health issues, researchers can ensure that valuable insights about safety and efficacy reach those most affected by misinformation.

In conclusion, understanding scientific consensus encompasses its formation process, its significance in guiding health decisions, and the challenges posed by misinformation. As we navigate the complex landscape of health claims—particularly those surrounding alternative remedies like apricot seeds—the importance of scientifically validated information cannot be overstated. By fortifying the public's understanding of scientific consensus, fostering critical thinking, and promoting open dialogue between the scientific community and the public, we can cultivate a culture of informed health choices. These choices must prioritize safety, efficacy, and community well-being, ensuring that individuals are empowered to navigate their health journeys responsibly.

15.4. Using Technology to Access Information

Using Technology to Access Information

In the rapidly evolving landscape of health communication, technology has become an indispensable tool for accessing and disseminating health information. Particularly in the context of alternative treatments such as apricot seeds—which have become subjects of both intrigue and controversy—leveraging technology effectively can empower individuals to make informed health choices. This subchapter explores various technological avenues that facilitate access to credible information, emphasizing the importance of utilizing these tools responsibly and thoughtfully.

The internet serves as the primary resource for many individuals seeking health information. A vast repository of knowledge awaits at one's fingertips, offering everything from anecdotal narratives to comprehensive academic articles. However, the sheer volume of content can be overwhelming, making discernment between credible resources and misinformation an essential skill. Accessing reliable health information directly from reputable websites—such as those of health organizations like the World Health Organization (WHO), the Centers for Disease Control and Prevention (CDC), and other esteemed medical institutions—should be prioritized. These platforms often provide scientifically vetted resources that can guide individuals in navigating claims surrounding alternative treatments, such as those regarding apricot seeds.

Furthermore, digital health literacy programs are emerging as pivotal initiatives aimed at educating the public on how to evaluate health claims critically. These programs teach individuals how to assess the credibility of sources, recognize red flags in health claims, and question the motivations behind certain narratives. By arming people with these skills, technology can transform the way health information is consumed. Workshops, webinars, and interactive online courses can provide practical training aimed at enhancing health literacy, making it easier for individuals to access and interpret health information confidently.

In addition to these educational resources, the development of mobile applications has revolutionized the way individuals manage their health. Various apps provide symptom checkers, medication reminders, nutritional guidance, and platforms for tracking health data. Topics related to alternative remedies can also be explored through these applications, which can offer balanced perspectives on their efficacy and risks. For example, an app might provide users with insights into the scientific literature concerning apricot seeds, juxtaposing anecdotal success stories with documented risks, thereby facilitating informed decision-making.

The impact of social media cannot be overstated in the realm of healthcare. Social media platforms have become arenas for sharing health-related information and experiences. Campaigns that promote accurate health messaging on platforms like Instagram, Facebook, and Twitter can reach vast audiences, increasing awareness about the potential risks of alternative treatments like apricot seeds. By creating engaging graphics, concise videos, and easy-to-understand infographics, public health organizations can leverage social media to dispel misconceptions and guide individuals towards evidence-based practices.

Moreover, integrating technology into healthcare delivery through telemedicine has transformed patient access to medical consultations. Patients seeking advice about alternative treatments can connect with healthcare providers remotely, receiving personalized guidance that considers their individual health circumstances. This direct engagement fosters dialogue about the safety and efficacy of various options, ensuring that patients receive accurate information while still exploring their preferences.

Collaborations between tech experts and health professionals can enhance the effectiveness of digital health initiatives. Tech professionals possess the tools and expertise to develop innovative platforms for health communication, creating user-friendly interfaces that facilitate user engagement. Health professionals can guide the design of these tools to ensure that they address the unique needs of patients and align with evidence-based practices. By utilizing the strengths of both fields, health communication efforts can achieve both clarity and effectiveness.

Looking to the future, the ongoing advancements in artificial intelligence (AI) and data analytics technology hold tremendous potential for revolutionizing health information accessibility. AI can assist in analyzing vast datasets to identify patterns relevant to public health trends, uncovering insights about the dissemination of misinformation and the public's engagement with health narratives. Additionally, machine learning algorithms can refine the way individuals search for health-related content, directing them towards reliable sources and facilitating more informed health decisions.

While technology provides powerful tools for accessing information, it must be coupled with a commitment to ethical considerations in health communication. Transparency regarding data use and privacy remains paramount, ensuring that individuals feel safe while accessing health resources. Furthermore, maintaining a critical lens on the information technology landscape is vital to prevent the unregulated spread of misinformation, which can lead individuals to pursue unsafe alternatives.

In summary, technology has the potential to reshape the conversation surrounding health information access, offering individuals powerful resources to navigate complex health narratives, including those surrounding alternative treatments like apricot seeds. By prioritizing credible sources, enhancing digital health literacy, leveraging social media, and promoting transparency and ethical practices, we can empower individuals to make well-informed health decisions. The journey towards a more informed public rests upon the effective collaboration between technology and healthcare, ensuring that the future of health information access remains rooted in evidence, safety, and empowerment.

15.5. Creating Personal Health Databases

Creating a personal health database can play a pivotal role in supporting one's health journey, especially in the context of nuanced discussions surrounding health choices like the consumption of apricot seeds. As individuals take charge of their health decisions, having a structured, reliable repository of personal health information can enhance understanding, improve communication with healthcare providers, and empower informed decision-making. This subchapter will explore the essential components of a personal health database, its significance, and actionable steps for its implementation.

At its core, a personal health database is a systematic compilation of one's health information that can include medical history, treatment regimens, laboratory results, medications, allergies, and lifestyle choices. This database can serve as a powerful tool for self-management, allowing individuals to track their health history, identify trends, and make informed choices about their healthcare. The ability to access this consolidated information readily can streamline discussions with healthcare providers, ensuring that individuals present a comprehensive overview of their health status when seeking advice.

One critical aspect of a personal health database is its role in documenting medical history. This includes any past illnesses, surgeries, and treatments undertaken, along with relevant family medical history. By compiling this information, individuals create a narrative of their health journey that can help healthcare providers better understand their current needs. This is particularly important when discussing potential risks associated with alternative treatments like apricot seeds. When patients can share their complete medical history, including any prior use of alternative therapies, it allows providers to offer tailored advice based on individual circumstances.

Tracking current and past medications is another essential component of a personal health database. Many people manage multiple prescriptions and supplements concurrently, which can complicate treatment regimens. Documenting medication details—such as dosages, frequency, and reasons for use—enables individuals to monitor changes, assess effectiveness, and communicate with healthcare providers about any interactions or side effects experienced. This is particularly relevant when discussing the appeal of alternative treatments, as the informed use of herbs and supplements—including apricot seeds—requires careful consideration of how they interact with conventional medications.

Furthermore, maintaining a record of laboratory results and diagnostic tests is important in creating a holistic view of one's health. Having easy access to test results can facilitate discussions between patients and providers, providing a framework for monitoring disease progress or response to treatments. As individuals explore their options for cancer treatment—whether through conventional means or alternative approaches—being able to reference their lab results can empower them to make informed decisions based on their unique health contexts.

Incorporating lifestyle choices into a personal health database is also beneficial in promoting overall wellness. Individuals can track dietary habits, exercise routines, mental well-being, sleep patterns, and other lifestyle factors that contribute to their health. This information helps individuals understand how these components interact with their medical conditions, influencing choices regarding alternative treatments. For example, those drawn to apricot seeds may reflect on their overall health, lifestyle habits, and responses to alternative remedies documented over time.

Creating a personal health database can be initiated through various tools, such as electronic health record (EHR) applications, health trackers, or even traditional pen-and-paper methods. Many mobile health applications allow individuals to input information about their health, medications, and symptoms, while also providing educational resources that encourage informed decision-making. It's critical for individuals to ensure that any digital applications used comply with data privacy standards, safeguarding personal information while promoting accessibility.

Moreover, the process of maintaining a health database should be seen as an ongoing commitment. Regular updates are essential to ensure that the information presented remains relevant and accurate. Individuals should establish a routine of inputting new information during healthcare visits, particularly when discussing alternative treatments or when any changes arise in their health status. This commitment fosters a proactive approach to health management, encouraging individuals to engage in their care continually.

In conclusion, creating a personal health database offers numerous benefits for individuals navigating health choices, especially concerning alternative treatments like apricot seeds. Documenting medical history, tracking medications, recording lab results, and incorporating lifestyle factors all contribute to a comprehensive view of one's health. This approach empowers individuals to engage in informed discussions with healthcare providers, ensuring that decisions reflect both personal experiences and scientific evidence. As health decisions become increasingly complex, cultivating a personal health database is a vital step toward effective health management, promoting safety, efficacy, and well-being throughout one's health journey.

16. Future Perspectives: Science, Society, and Health

16.1. Innovations in Medicine

Innovations in Medicine represent the culmination of progress in research, technology, and the understanding of human health. This subchapter serves as a holistic exploration of the current landscape of medical advancements and their implications for the future of healthcare, particularly in the context of cancer treatment and alternative therapies such as apricot seeds.

The rapid pace of technological advancements has reshaped the way healthcare is delivered. Innovations like precision medicine, which tailors treatments based on an individual's genetic makeup, have transformed the landscape of cancer treatment. Precision oncology seeks to identify the specific mutations driving a patient's cancer, allowing for targeted therapies that are designed to attack those specific alterations. This personalized approach not only enhances treatment efficacy but also minimizes the risk of side effects by sparing healthy cells.

Moreover, the advent of immunotherapy marks a significant breakthrough in cancer treatment. By harnessing the body's immune system to combat malignant cells, immunotherapy has the potential to change the prognosis for patients with certain types of cancer. Treatments such as checkpoint inhibitors have demonstrated remarkable success in previously untreatable cancers, showcasing the potential of innovations to redefine the boundaries of medical intervention.

Biotechnology continues to thrive as a field driving innovation in medicine. The development of CAR T-cell therapy exemplifies this trend. By genetically modifying a patient's own T-cells to recognize and attack cancer cells, this innovative approach has emerged as a powerful weapon in the fight against hematologic malignancies. The success of CAR T-cell therapy highlights the incredible potential of biotechnology to reshape our understanding of treatment options, moving us away from traditional methodologies toward more dynamic, individualized therapies.

The integration of artificial intelligence (AI) into healthcare systems promises to enhance diagnostics and treatment planning. AI algorithms can analyze vast datasets from clinical studies, genomic sequences, and patient records, enabling healthcare providers to make informed decisions rapidly. Predictive analytics powered by AI can identify patients at risk for certain diseases, opening avenues for preventative care, early intervention, and overall improved health outcomes. As AI continues to evolve, its role in optimizing treatment protocols and streamlining the healthcare workflow emerges as a valuable asset.

Telemedicine has also revolutionized access to healthcare services, particularly during crises such as the COVID-19 pandemic. Remote consultations have not only provided continuity of care but have also broadened access to specialized care for individuals in underserved communities. As patients increasingly utilize telehealth for consultations, the incorporation of technology into healthcare delivery models ensures that individuals can seek advice from experts without geographical barriers. This development underscores the ongoing innovations aiming to create a more equitable healthcare landscape.

However, as we celebrate these advancements, ethical considerations remain paramount. The rapid integration of new technologies into medicine must be coupled with rigorous oversight to ensure patient safety, privacy, and the integrity of scientific research. The dialogue surrounding innovations in medicine must also address the disparities in access that persist, ensuring that evolving therapeutic options benefit all populations rather than exacerbating health inequities.

Moreover, public engagement and discourse surrounding medical innovations are essential. Health communication strategies must convey the potential benefits and risks of novel treatments accurately, allowing individuals to make informed choices grounded in evidence. In the context of alternative treatments like apricot seeds, it is vital that innovations in medicine are framed within a narrative that distinguishes them from sensationalized claims. Continuous education regarding scientific advancements—paired with public trust in healthcare professionals—can mitigate the lure of unverified remedies.

Ultimately, the future of medicine is a tapestry woven from advancements aimed at improving health outcomes while striving to ensure patient safety and ethical integrity. As we move forward, the focus should remain on fostering collaboration among healthcare professionals, researchers, policymakers, and the public. Together, we can build a healthcare environment that honors the incredible potential of innovations in medicine while promoting health equity, safety, and informed decision-making, ultimately reshaping the future of cancer treatment and the broader health landscape.

16.2. Anticipating Changes in Health Policy

Anticipating changes in health policy in relation to alternative treatments, particularly the use of apricot seeds as a purported cancer cure, is crucial for navigating the complexities of health communication and patient safety. The evolving landscape of healthcare necessitates an awareness of regulatory trends, public perception, and the integration of evidence-based practices to foster a comprehensive understanding of how health policies are likely to adapt over time.

Current health policies often reflect a growing recognition of the importance of regulating alternative treatments. The surge of interest in natural remedies and holistic health approaches has led to increased scrutiny of unverified claims, especially those associated with alternative therapies. As awareness regarding the potential dangers associated with unregulated treatments, such as apricot seeds, continues to grow, policymakers will likely prioritize the establishment of stricter regulations governing the marketing of such products. This evolution will be essential in protecting consumers from misleading information and ensuring that alternative treatments undergo the same rigorous evaluation as conventional therapies.

Moreover, as more individuals turn to alternative treatments, there is a pressing need for integrating these options within traditional healthcare frameworks. Policymakers may focus on fostering collaboration between conventional providers and practitioners of alternative medicine to create comprehensive treatment plans that consider both evidence-based practices and patient preferences. This integrative approach can benefit from continued dialogue and professional exchanges, ultimately prioritizing patient safety while supporting informed health choices.

Public perception of alternative treatments will also play a significant role in shaping future health policies. The narratives surrounding the appeal of natural remedies like apricot seeds are often rooted in emotional resonance, personal stories, and cultural beliefs. Policymakers should anticipate shifts in sociocultural attitudes toward health that favor holistic approaches and incorporate these trends in guiding regulatory efforts. This may involve the creation of educational campaigns that emphasize the significance of science-based health choices while acknowledging the psychological and cultural dimensions associated with alternative remedies.

Incorporating technology into health policy is another aspect to consider. As telehealth services proliferate, policymakers must adapt existing regulations to ensure that access to care is equitable while safeguarding patient data and privacy. The rise of digital health platforms offers opportunities to disseminate accurate information about alternative treatments, yet this also necessitates vigilance against the spread of misinformation online. Future policies may address the integration of digital health tools aimed at enhancing health literacy and empowering individuals to make informed decisions regarding their treatment options.

The importance of community engagement will be paramount in anticipating health policy changes surrounding alternative treatments. As diverse populations seek out healthcare solutions that align with their cultural values, policymakers must be responsive to these communities. Initiatives that promote the collaboration of public health organizations, community leaders, and healthcare providers can ensure that health policies are informed by the lived experiences and preferences of the populace.

Finally, continuous research will be a cornerstone as policymakers adapt health regulations to address the complexities of alternative treatments. As scientific understanding of the effects of alternative remedies evolves, monitoring the efficacy and safety of these treatments through robust research will inform policy revisions. Legislative bodies must remain adaptable, ready to respond to emerging evidence while also engaging the public in meaningful dialogues regarding health choices.

In conclusion, anticipating changes in health policy related to alternative treatments requires a multifaceted approach that incorporates regulatory awareness, public engagement, the evolution of public perception, technological integration, and continuous research. As the healthcare landscape shifts toward embracing integrative practices that respect patients' agency and preferences, it is critical that policymakers and healthcare professionals prioritize evidence-based approaches, ensuring that consumers receive comprehensive, safe, and effective care. By fostering a responsive and inclusive dialogue with communities, we can pave the way towards a healthcare system that truly values patient safety and informed decision-making in the coming years.

16.3. The Role of Community in Public Health

In exploring the role of community in public health, particularly in the context of alternative treatments such as the claims surrounding apricot seeds as a cancer cure, it becomes evident that community dynamics significantly influence health behavior, beliefs, and access to information. Healthy communities are characterized by strong communication networks, shared values, and a collective approach to understanding and addressing health concerns, all of which play crucial roles in shaping public health outcomes.

Communities serve as foundational units for disseminating health information and fostering dialogue on treatment choices. When individuals within a community discuss their health experiences and share stories—be they successes or challenges—these narratives can exert profound influences on collective beliefs about health interventions. In the case of apricot seeds, anecdotal testimonials praising their supposed benefits shape the local narrative, drawing individuals towards unverified remedies. However, when communities facilitate open discussions about the risks associated with these treatments, individuals may feel more empowered to seek out evidence-based alternatives.

The social network aspect cannot be underestimated. Friends, family members, and local leaders often serve as key influencers in shaping health behaviors. Community leaders can play a pivotal role in setting public health priorities and advocating for evidence-based practices, particularly in regions where traditional beliefs about natural remedies are deeply entrenched. Collaborative efforts among healthcare providers, public health officials, and community leaders can foster awareness and understanding of risks associated with treatments like apricot seeds, encouraging individuals to engage with reputable health sources rather than anecdotal claims.

Formal health education programs within communities also contribute to the dissemination of accurate health information. These initiatives can address common misconceptions and empower individuals to critically evaluate health claims they encounter. For instance, a community-focused campaign could educate individuals about the scientific consensus regarding apricot seeds while highlighting safe, evidence-based treatments. Workshops, public lectures, and health fairs serve as vital tools for delivering messages that prioritize health literacy and informed decision-making.

Furthermore, community engagement acts as a buffer against misinformation. When individuals are embedded within strong community networks, they are more likely to seek verification of health claims from trusted sources rather than relying solely on sensationalized stories circulating online. This vital role of a supportive community environment can help counterbalance the overwhelming tide of misinformation about alternative remedies.

Health disparities are another critical factor influenced by community dynamics. Marginalized communities often face barriers in accessing quality healthcare and reliable health information, leading to heightened susceptibility to alternative treatments. Public health initiatives that thoughtfully engage with underserved populations can help dismantle these barriers, providing education and access to resources that promote equity in health. In this sense, community empowerment becomes an integral aspect of addressing health challenges and improving overall public health outcomes.

An important outlet for leveraging community influence lies in advocacy. Communities can form coalitions to champion health rights and push for policy changes that prioritize evidence-based practices while providing protection against misleading health claims. For instance, advocacy groups can raise awareness about potential dangers associated with unverified treatments, urging policymakers to implement rigorous regulations around their marketing and promotion.

In essence, the role of community in public health is essential for fostering informed health choices that recognize and respect individual beliefs while grounding discussions in scientific understanding. Engaging communities, prioritizing health education, and bolstering local support systems enhances resilience against misinformation and empowers individuals to make sound health decisions.

In summation, the interplay between community dynamics and public health is critical, especially in addressing issues centered around alternative treatments like apricot seeds. By fostering a culture of trust, communication, and informed decision-making, communities can work towards creating an environment that prioritizes health and well-being, leading to improved public health outcomes and a better quality of life for all individuals. It is through concerted community efforts that the conversation surrounding alternative and conventional treatments can be shaped, nurturing a more holistic approach to public health challenges in the contemporary landscape.

16.4. The Legacy of 21st Century Medical Breakthroughs

In the realm of medical advancements, the 21st century has been remarkably transformative, marked by a sequence of breakthroughs that have shifted paradigms in cancer treatment and overall healthcare. As we evaluate the legacy of these medical breakthroughs, it's essential to consider not only the achievements themselves but also the broader implications of these innovations for public health and individual wellness in the context of alternative treatments such as apricot seeds.

One of the most significant features of the medical advancements of this century is the shift towards personalized medicine. This approach tailors treatment to the individual characteristics of each patient— particularly their genetic makeup. Advances in genomic sequencing and biomarker identification have paved the way for targeted therapies that can effectively combat cancer while minimizing side effects. For instance, drugs developed to target specific mutations found in tumors have shown remarkable efficacy, ushering in a new era of hope for patients diagnosed with forms of cancer that were once deemed intractable. This revolution in targeted treatment emphasizes the necessity of grounding health decisions in evidence-based practices while illuminating the ineffective nature of alternative remedies lacking scientific backing, such as apricot seeds.

Moreover, the era of immunotherapy represents another major leap forward. By enhancing the body's immune response against cancer cells, therapies like checkpoint inhibitors have radically changed treatment protocols for various types of cancer. This breakthrough not only improves outcomes for some patients but also highlights a more profound understanding of cancer biology—shifting focus from merely eliminating tumors to reactivating the body's natural defenses. The successes seen in these innovative treatments contrast sharply with unverified claims overlooking the complexity of cancer treatment, further illustrating the importance of quality evidence in guiding patient health decisions.

The integration of technology into healthcare, particularly through telemedicine, also stands out as a crucial aspect of 21st-century breakthroughs. The COVID-19 pandemic accelerated the adoption of telehealth services, demonstrating their potential to improve access to care, especially for individuals residing in remote or underserved areas. By fostering seamless interaction between patients and providers, telemedicine nurtures a holistic approach to health management grounded in continual care and support. This technological evolution underscores the need for open communication between patients and healthcare professionals—particularly when navigating potential unregulated alternatives like apricot seeds.

However, the enhancements in medical research and technology come with commensurate responsibilities. As much as advancements offer opportunities for improved patient outcomes, they also compel us to confront the challenges of misinformation and the oversimplification of treatment narratives. The elevation of personal testimonials as valid proof of efficacy often overshadows the critical nature of empirical evidence. Thus, the legacy of these breakthroughs must encompass a commitment to lifelong health education and a drive to dispel myths surrounding alternative treatments.

Furthermore, the legacies of today's medical breakthroughs extend beyond individual patient outcomes. The ethical dimensions and societal implications of innovations in medicine provoke essential discussions surrounding equitable access to care, the underscoring of diverse patient perspectives, and the promotion of safe health practices. Policymakers have a pivotal role to play in shaping health policies that prioritize safety, support evidence-based practice, and mitigate the risks of promoting unverified treatments.

As we prognosticate the future of cancer treatment, several factors become paramount. Anticipating advancements in treatment research, particularly in integrating innovation with historical practices, offers insights into achieving a holistic framework for healthcare. Collaboration across disciplines, active patient engagement, and continuous assessment of alternative treatments can guide the trajectory of medical breakthroughs, harnessing the full potential of contemporary innovations while ensuring the safety of individuals encountering unproven therapies.

In conclusion, the legacy of 21st-century medical breakthroughs embodies profound advancements in treatment and understanding, shaping the landscape of health and wellness. However, it also highlights the essential responsibility to ground health practices in evidenced knowledge. As society whole, we must strive for a future where informed health choices prevail above the perils of misinformation and false promises. By championing a commitment to health advocacy, fostering community dialogue, and promoting equitable access to information, we can pave the way for a healthier, more informed world where individual agency in health choices harmonizes with scientific integrity. As we reflect on the lessons learned and anticipate future changes, let us reaffirm our dedication to advancing medicine, emphasizing informed decision-making, and cultivating a sustainable health future for generations to come.

16.5. Speculating on the Future of Cancer Treatment

As we contemplate the future of cancer treatment, there are several trends and developments on the horizon that signal meaningful change in the way we approach this complex, multifaceted disease. The ongoing evolution of research methodologies, technological innovations, and integrative approaches will all play crucial roles in shaping future cancer therapies. The prospects for more personalized, effective treatments are not only the outcomes of scientific inquiry but also reflections of an increasingly informed public that values agency in health decisions.

One significant movement is the transition toward more personalized cancer therapies. Advances in genomics and molecular biology have opened new frontiers in our understanding of cancer biology, allowing for treatments that are historically tailored to the unique genetic makeup of individual tumors. This precision medicine approach —where therapies are matched to the specific genetic alterations present in a patient's cancer—will likely become increasingly standard practice. For instance, targeted therapies that alter the biological pathways that drive cancer growth may replace more generalized treatment paradigms, enhancing efficacy while minimizing side effects.

Similarly, the growing field of immunotherapy represents a bold new frontier in how we approach cancer treatment. Innovative therapies that harness the body's immune system to detect and eradicate cancer cells showcase promising outcomes where traditional treatments have faltered. Research continues to emerge from clinical trials exploring varying combinations of immunotherapies, allowing oncologists to establish more individualized treatment regimens that resonate with patients' unique needs and conditions.

Moreover, technology will play a vital role in how healthcare is delivered. The integration of artificial intelligence (AI) and machine learning into oncology research and practice offers the potential to analyze vast amounts of patient data and enhance diagnostic accuracy. These innovations can help identify treatment pathways based on real-time patient data analytics, ultimately improving patient outcomes. Similarly, the use of telemedicine will likely continue to grow, breaking down barriers to access and allowing patients in remote areas to seek timely consultations with cancer specialists.

Additionally, there is a growing recognition of the need for comprehensive support systems that address not only the physiological aspects of cancer but also the psychological and emotional ramifications of a cancer diagnosis. Integrative approaches that consider diet, lifestyle changes, and mental health alongside conventional therapy are becoming increasingly common. Programs that facilitate holistic care provide patients with the tools to navigate both their treatment and their overall well-being, empowering them to make informed choices throughout their cancer journey.

As we reflect on the importance of public health education and proactive communication, it becomes clear that there must be a strong emphasis on combating misinformation surrounding alternative treatments. The narrative surrounding cancer treatment, particularly regarding options like apricot seeds, reinforces the necessity of scientific literacy. Educating patients and communities about the risks associated with unregulated therapies while emphasizing sound, evidence-based alternatives will establish a healthier public discourse about treatment options.

The implications of these developments extend beyond individual patient experiences; they also underscore the importance of health equity. As healthcare practitioners and policymakers advocate for access to innovative treatments, it is imperative to ensure that all populations benefit equitably from advancements in cancer treatment. This includes addressing disparities in healthcare access, affordability, and knowledge.

In conclusion, speculating on the future of cancer treatment unveils a landscape teeming with possibilities shaped by innovation, personalized medicine, technological integration, and holistic approaches to care. As we move forward, there is a collective responsibility to prioritize patient safety, educate the public, and promote evidence-based practices while respecting individual beliefs and values.

The pathway to a healthier world depends on our commitment to informed health advocacy and open dialogue for change. By championing scientific literacy and enhancing public engagement, we can create an informed society that values sound evidence above sensationalized claims.

Ultimately, the future of cancer treatment lies in advancements that enhance our approach to healing—embracing a holistic understanding of health that empowers individuals while leaving room for incorporating culturally relevant practices. As we navigate these transformations, let us strive for a sustainable health future that prioritizes equity, informed choice, and the well-being of all individuals in their health journeys.

17. Concluding Thoughts: Wise Health Choices for Lifelong Wellness

17.1. Summarizing Key Lessons

In the subchapter 'Summarizing Key Lessons', we bring together the insights and experiences discussed throughout the book, distilling key takeaways that can inform and empower individuals in their health journeys. The exploration of apricot seeds as a potential cancer remedy serves as a poignant case study highlighting the dangers of misinformation while illuminating the central tenets of informed decision-making, critical thinking, and responsible health practices.

The first key lesson underscores the critical importance of grounding health choices in credible, evidence-based information. Throughout the discussion, we have examined how the allure of alternative remedies can often overshadow scientific consensus, leading individuals towards choices that may pose significant risks. This highlights the necessity of discernment and the proactive evaluation of health claims, particularly those related to alternative treatments. As demonstrated by the narratives surrounding apricot seeds, anecdotal evidence may resonate emotionally but cannot substitute for rigorous scientific validation and professional medical guidance.

Moreover, the role of health literacy cannot be overstated. The ability to access, read, and critically assess health information empowers individuals to navigate the complexities of their health decisions effectively. We have seen that enhancing health literacy through community education, digital platforms, and proactive engagement can help combat misinformation and promote responsible health choices. Such initiatives equip individuals with the tools to evaluate the credibility of sources, recognize potential biases, and ultimately cultivate a culture of informed health decision-making.

Another important takeaway is the value of fostering open dialogues that bridge the gap between healthcare professionals and communities. Collaborative efforts that involve public health advocates, healthcare providers, and patients create an environment conducive to empowerment and transparency. By promoting inclusive conversations that honor cultural beliefs while stressing scientific evidence, we can enhance understanding and facilitate informed discussions surrounding health narratives, as illustrated by the misleading claims related to apricot seeds.

The impact of personal narratives cannot be overlooked, as they often play a significant role in shaping public perception of health practices. While survivor stories and testimonials can inspire hope and resilience, it is crucial to contextualize these narratives within a framework of scientific inquiry. Recognizing the emotional weight of personal experiences while emphasizing the limitations of anecdotal evidence enables us to honor individual journeys while advocating for evidence-based practices that prioritize patient safety.

Finally, the importance of community engagement and access to reliable resources stands as a key lesson. Libraries, digital archives, and public health campaigns play a vital role in disseminating accurate information and fostering health literacy. Through equitable access to credible health data and resources, we can empower communities to make informed choices while bridging gaps in knowledge and addressing disparities in healthcare access.

In conclusion, as we summarize these key lessons, we are reminded that the journey toward wise health choices requires a multifaceted approach rooted in evidence, education, and collaborative dialogue. By prioritizing scientific inquiry, embracing health literacy, and promoting community engagement, we can build a healthier society that values informed decision-making and advances public health. The ongoing commitment to understanding the complexities of health narratives and promoting safety will serve as the foundation for individuals to navigate their health journeys with confidence and empowerment in an era marked by both hope and uncertainty.

17.2. The Path to a Healthier World

In the quest for a healthier world, we must recognize the intricate interplay between knowledge, empowerment, and community engagement. The narratives surrounding alternative treatments, particularly those as contentious as apricot seeds purported to combat cancer, unveil the broader implications of misinformation and the resulting need for transformative changes in public health communication.

One of the most critical aspects of this journey is the commitment to personal health advocacy. Individuals must take active roles in their health journeys, seeking out credible information, questioning misleading claims, and understanding the risks associated with unverified remedies. This commitment extends beyond personal health choices; it involves advocating for informed decision-making within one's community and fostering a culture that values evidence-based practices. Emphasizing health literacy equips individuals with the tools to critically evaluate health information, reinforcing their ability to navigate complex narratives surrounding health topics.

Moreover, our path toward a healthier world is marked by the necessity of inviting open dialogues for change. Engaging with diverse perspectives—especially those from marginalized communities—enables us to understand the cultural beliefs and experiences that shape health narratives. By fostering collaborative conversations between healthcare professionals, community leaders, and public health advocates, we can dismantle barriers of mistrust and misinformation. This dialogue must prioritize education and transparency, empowering individuals to make informed choices that respect their values while grounding discussions in science.

The role of community in these conversations cannot be understated. Communities serve as vital networks where people share resources, support one another, and collectively address health challenges. By leveraging these networks, public health initiatives can engage with individuals on a more personal level, leading to increased awareness and understanding of important health topics. These initiatives should emphasize the significance of accurate information, dispelling myths around alternative treatments and reinforcing the importance of seeking evidence-based options.

As we look toward our sustainable health future, we must commit to ongoing research and innovation in medicine. The landscape of healthcare is ever-evolving, and future breakthroughs in cancer treatment and other areas will continue to shape public health. By advocating for science-driven policies, encouraging interdisciplinary collaboration, and investing in community health education, we can create an environment that prioritizes safety, efficacy, and informed health choices for all individuals.

In conclusion, the path to a healthier world necessitates a multi-faceted approach rooted in personal commitment to health advocacy, community engagement, and open dialogue. By prioritizing these values and embracing the principles of evidence-based practices, we can cultivate an informed society resilient against misinformation. The journey towards empowering individuals and communities will ensure that public health flourishes, creating a landscape marked by safety, understanding, and well-being for everyone involved.

By fostering a culture of transparency, collaboration, and education, we pave the way for a future where individuals can navigate their health journeys with confidence, resilience, and informed decision-making at the forefront of their choices. As we commit to these principles, we can transform the discourse surrounding health into one that is constructive, empowering, and centered around lifelong wellness.

17.3. Commitment to Personal Health Advocacy

Commitment to Personal Health Advocacy represents an essential dimension in navigating the intricate landscape of health information, particularly in a world characterized by a plethora of alternative treatment narratives. The pursuit of health advocacy is particularly crucial when considering topics rife with misinformation, such as the claims surrounding apricot seeds as potential cancer cures. This sub-chapter delves deep into the significance of personal health advocacy, outlining its importance, strategies for implementation, and its role in promoting informed decision-making and patient empowerment.

At the core of personal health advocacy lies the principle of informed choice. Individuals have the right to understand their health conditions, the treatments available, and the evidence supporting these options. This empowerment starts with education. By being well-informed, individuals can actively engage in discussions about their health with healthcare professionals, making choices that align with their values and preferences. When faced with claims about unverified alternative treatments, such as apricot seeds, knowing the risks and benefits becomes crucial for steering clear of potentially harmful decisions.

Building a commitment to personal health advocacy includes fostering critical thinking skills and encouraging individuals to question the validity of information they encounter. The current digital landscape is flooded with competing health claims, particularly related to natural remedies. By cultivating a mindset of inquiry, individuals can proactively assess the credibility of sources, recognizing whether claims are supported by scientific evidence or are merely anecdotal. This discernment forms the bedrock of effective health advocacy, where individuals become not just passive recipients of information but active participants in their health journeys.

Individuals should also embrace their role in advocating not only for themselves but also for others within their communities. Engaging in conversations about health practices, sharing accurate information, and supporting peers in navigating their health journeys contributes to an environment where informed health choices flourish. By disseminating knowledge regarding the risks associated with alternative treatments, such as the potential dangers relating to apricot seeds, advocates can help safeguard their communities from misinformation.

Additionally, establishing a relationship with healthcare providers is vital in the commitment to personal health advocacy. Patients should feel empowered to ask questions and seek second opinions, thereby promoting a culture of open dialogue in healthcare settings. This collaborative approach not only encourages transparency but also fosters trust between patients and providers, enhancing the overall healthcare experience. When individuals feel that they can express their concerns regarding treatment options—whether conventional or alternative—they are more likely to make informed, safe health decisions.

Moreover, community engagement plays a significant role in promoting health advocacy. By participating in community health initiatives or workshops, individuals can access valuable resources, information, and support networks. This collaboration can take various forms, including public health campaigns that address misinformation regarding alternative treatments, leading to widespread awareness of potential risks. Health fairs, educational seminars, and outreach programs can foster environments in which community members are empowered to engage in discussions about their health and practices.

The evolving narrative of personal health advocacy must also recognize and incorporate the rich historical contexts and cultural beliefs that inform individuals' perspectives on health and wellness. Respecting these backgrounds promotes stronger connections, allowing advocates to navigate health discussions more effectively. By acknowledging and exploring the emotional resonance of natural remedies, advocates can guide discussions that balance personal values with the need for credible, evidence-based health practices.

As the healthcare landscape continues to shift, individuals' commitment to personal health advocacy must adapt accordingly. Emerging technologies can provide innovative methods for engaging in health promotion, offering tools for tracking health metrics, researching credible information, and connecting with healthcare professionals virtually. Utilizing digital platforms responsibly can enhance individual agency while navigating health decisions, ensuring that choices are rooted in evidence and safety.

Ultimately, the commitment to personal health advocacy involves recognizing the significant power individuals have in shaping their health destinies. By fostering critical thinking, engaging in open dialogue with healthcare providers and peers, and participating in community initiatives, individuals can navigate the complex terrain of health information with confidence. As we delve deeper into discussions regarding alternative treatments like apricot seeds, advocating for safety, efficacy, and informed decisions will be essential in ensuring that health choices are rooted in knowledge rather than misinformation.

In conclusion, the commitment to personal health advocacy encapsulates the aspiration to empower individuals with the knowledge and skills necessary to navigate the complexities of health choices responsibly. By promoting informed decision-making and fostering open discussions about health narratives, we can transform the discourse surrounding health practices, ultimately paving the way for a healthier society grounded in evidence-based solutions. As this commitment grows stronger, it propels individuals toward lifelong wellness, ensuring that they are equipped to make wise health choices in an ever-changing landscape.

17.4. Inviting Open Dialogues for Change

Inviting open dialogues for change stands as a pivotal concept in navigating the complex landscape of health choices, particularly in the context of alternative treatments such as apricot seeds purported to heal cancer. This subchapter emphasizes the importance of fostering inclusive conversations that engage diverse voices, promote transparency, and facilitate collaborative learning in the pursuit of informed health decisions. The necessity of inviting such dialogues is underscored by the growing prevalence of misinformation, emotional narratives, and the urgent need for safe, evidence-based practices in healthcare.

At the heart of inviting open dialogues is the recognition that health issues are deeply personal and often laden with emotional weight. Individuals facing serious health challenges, such as a cancer diagnosis, can feel overwhelmed by the myriad treatment options and information available. In these moments, creating safe spaces for dialogue becomes essential—spaces where individuals can express their fears, share their stories, and navigate the uncertainty surrounding their health choices. Such dialogues foster a sense of community, ensuring that individuals do not feel isolated in their health journeys.

Furthermore, open dialogues that incorporate diverse perspectives also enhance our understanding of health issues across cultural contexts. Different communities bring unique beliefs, traditions, and experiences that inform their approaches to health and wellness. Engaging with these narratives allows for a more holistic understanding of health challenges while fostering mutual respect and learning among individuals. For instance, when discussing alternative treatments like apricot seeds, it is essential to acknowledge the cultural significance some individuals may attribute to these remedies while also providing clear information about the associated risks.

As healthcare becomes increasingly complex and technology-driven, promoting open dialogues necessitates leveraging digital platforms effectively. Online forums, social media, and virtual community spaces can serve as venues for individuals to engage in discussions about health choices and shared experiences. These platforms represent a unique opportunity to connect individuals from diverse backgrounds, facilitating dialogues that address health concerns while providing evidence-based information. By actively participating in these digital spaces, health professionals can counteract misinformation and help shape public discourse around alternative treatments.

Moreover, fostering dialogues opens avenues for collaboration between healthcare providers and patients. By encouraging individuals to voice their questions and concerns, healthcare professionals can better understand their patients' values and motivations. This collaboration enhances the shared decision-making process, ensuring that individuals feel empowered in their treatment choices. In the case of discussions surrounding apricot seeds, engaging with patients about their interests can lead to constructive conversations that emphasize safety and efficacy.

Additionally, inviting open dialogues is essential for addressing the psychological factors that influence health decisions. The emotional resonance tied to narratives—both personal and shared—can significantly impact an individual's perception of treatment options. By fostering a culture of dialogue that validates the emotional weight of health decisions, health advocates can better equip individuals with the tools to evaluate claims critically and responsibly.

As we navigate this complex landscape, the role of advocacy organizations in facilitating open dialogues cannot be overlooked. These organizations represent vital links between individuals and healthcare providers, amplifying the voices of patients while promoting education and awareness. Initiatives focused on engaging communities in collaborative discussions around health challenge the status quo and support informed decision-making. In this way, advocates can bridge gaps that may exist between traditional medical practices and alternative treatments, fostering understanding and cooperation.

In conclusion, inviting open dialogues for change is essential in cultivating an informed public willing to engage in discussions around alternative treatments such as apricot seeds. By fostering inclusive conversations that honor diverse perspectives, leverage digital platforms, and promote collaboration with healthcare professionals, we can empower individuals to make informed health decisions that prioritize safety and efficacy. As we strive for transparency and understanding in these discussions, we can pave the way for a future where informed choices and open discourse reign, fostering trust and collaboration among healthcare providers, advocates, and the communities they serve.

Through a commitment to inviting dialogues, we can reshape the narrative surrounding health choices, ensuring that personal experiences are respected while still prioritizing a foundation of scientific inquiry. In doing so, we contribute to a sustainable health future that values informed decision-making and holistic well-being for all individuals.

17.5. Towards a Sustainable Health Future

In contemplating the future of health practices, particularly in the context of alternative treatments, a sustainable approach is paramount. The narrative surrounding apricot seeds as a remedy for cancer serves as a guiding case study, highlighting the intersection of hope, misinformation, and the critical need for informed decision-making. As we move forward, the emphasis must be on fostering an environment that values evidence-based practices, encourages open communication, and empowers individuals to navigate their health journeys responsibly.

The sustainable health future requires a commitment to education and awareness, with a focus on enhancing health literacy across diverse populations. Initiatives that promote understanding of how to evaluate health claims critically, discern credible sources, and recognize the potential risks associated with unverified treatments are essential. As misinformation proliferates in digital spaces, equipping individuals with the tools necessary to navigate this complex landscape becomes imperative. Health campaigns should emphasize the importance of consulting healthcare professionals and seeking second opinions when considering alternative remedies.

Moreover, integrating community engagement into health initiatives is crucial for creating an informed society. By inviting diverse voices into the conversation, we can build a collective understanding of health issues that respects cultural beliefs while promoting evidence-based practices. This approach fosters trust and collaboration, empowering communities to engage in discussions about their health choices. When addressing the allure of natural remedies like apricot seeds, recognizing these cultural dynamics can nuance conversations and encourage individuals to consider the broader implications of their health decisions.

Technological advancements also play a vital role in shaping the future of health communication. By utilizing digital platforms to disseminate accurate health information and engage with audiences, public health organizations can counteract misinformation and promote informed choices. Innovative tools such as mobile applications, telemedicine, and online health resources enhance accessibility and allow individuals to actively participate in discussions surrounding their health. As technology continues to evolve, it presents opportunities to strengthen connections between healthcare providers and individuals, ultimately fostering a culture of shared responsibility in health decision-making.

The future of health also hinges on the ethical considerations surrounding the promotion of alternative treatments. As we engage with the stories of individuals drawn to natural remedies, there remains a responsibility to prioritize safety and efficacy. This calls for a collaborative effort between healthcare professionals, researchers, policymakers, and community advocates to foster an environment that emphasizes responsible messaging and equitable healthcare access. Regulatory measures will play a crucial role in ensuring that alternative treatments are subject to the same scrutiny as conventional medicine, protecting individuals from misleading claims while allowing for informed exploration of diverse health options.

In conclusion, towards a sustainable health future, the imperative of informed decision-making must remain paramount. By promoting health literacy, engaging communities, leveraging technology, and maintaining ethical vigilance, we can create an environment that champions evidence-based practices while respecting individual beliefs. The ongoing exploration of narratives surrounding alternative treatments like apricot seeds calls for a commitment to transparency, collaboration, and education—ensuring that individuals navigate their health journeys with confidence, knowledge, and empowerment.

As we advocate for a future where informed choices are the norm, we must harness the full potential of our scientific advancements and ethical commitments to health, paving the way for a healthier society. Together, by prioritizing safety and efficacy over sensational claims, we can cultivate a sustainable health future that uplifts all individuals, ensuring that wellness is within reach and grounded in knowledge.

Printed in Great Britain
by Amazon

57856991R00119